Striving

for

Imprefection

per

SCOTT "Q" MARCUS

THINspirational Columnist and Recovering Perfectionist

A sixth year of

^52 Inspirational
Playful Columns
on Living Well,
Changing Habits,
and Other Acts of Faith

Striving for Imperfection
Volume 6

© 2012 by
Scott Marcus

ISBN: 978-1468124071
Printed in the United States of America

Printed in the United States of America

For additional copies of this book, or to hire Scott "Q" Marcus for speaking,
training, consulting or workshops, call 707.442.6243
or scottq@scottqmarcus.com.

To get past what holds you or your business back,
go to www.ThisTimeIMeanIt.com
or
or www.ScottQMarcus.com

03.13.12

During this past year, I was hit by a car while riding my bicycle. The outpouring of support from strangers and friends was one of the most spiritually moving events of my life (although I do not recommend that as a way to have your faith enhanced).

This volume is dedicated to the people who helped me during — and after — my accident.

You will never know how much it meant.

TABLE OF CONTENTS

Contents

Striving

for

Imprefection

per

SCOTT "Q" MARCUS

THINspirational Columnist and Recovering Perfectionist

A sixth year of

^52 Inspirational
Playful Columns
on Living Well,
Changing Habits,
and Other Acts of Faith

RECOLLECTIONS FROM FIVE YEARS

I beg a bit of personal indulgence.

On my hard drive exists a folder named "My Column." Within it reside five sub-folders: "Year One," "Year Two," … through "Year Five," where I save every column I wrote during that corresponding year. While preparing for today's article, I noted that the footer in the "Year Five" directory says "52 documents," meaning I have completed half a decade. This will be "document one" in the sub-folder named "Year Six."

When I began this adventure, the editor of the Eureka Times-Standard, my hometown newspaper and the first to sign on; "we'll go for a month and monitor the reaction." After four weeks, I heard nothing. Figuring "no news is good news," I continued to send in my columns; still no feedback. It appeared every week, page one in the Health section like clockwork, so I assumed all was hunky dory. Yet, I figured I better call to confirm.

"Charles," I said, "It's Scott." (He didn't say "Scott who?" That's a good sign.) "You said we'd try the column for a month. It's been two. How's it going?"

"Oh yeah," he replied, "To be honest, we haven't heard anything…"

My heart sunk; my career was over.

"… which is good," he continued. "Usually if the readers don't like it, we hear about it in no time. No one's called to complain, that's good. Let's keep going."

"Cool! I'm a columnist!" I thought, soon I'll be hanging out with George Will or Thomas Friedman at fancy-columnist-guy conventions. I'll be hob-knobbing with the rich and famous. I was writing my Pulitzer acceptance speech already. It'll be so easy. Write about what I know; weight loss. I can regale the dieting public for years with somewhat humorous, intellectually keen, emotionally significant, well-crafted narratives. Of course, it hasn't always been that way; and, as with most of life, it has been quite the learning experience.

Do not believe the reports that the newspaper industry is dead. I can assure you, based on my experiences, it is very much alive — and an extremely potent force to boot. From the one-inch photograph at the top of this column, I have been recognized in several cities. I'm wandering about caught up in my life, when a reader approaches me, usually at a restaurant, and says, "Is that on your diet?" or "Should you be eating that?" (Note: I am not watching what you eat; please don't watch what I eat.)

Yet, more folks have inspected my grocery cart in supermarkets than have inspected my luggage in airports. I unwittingly started an unintended hub-bub when someone read the online version of my column where I was lamenting having a hard time locating low-calorie food in New Orleans. (I thought I was being cute; apparently I insulted everyone south of the Mason-Dixon line; who's to know?) On the other hand, I'm always flattered when someone tells me, "I cut out your article and mailed it to my sister; she really needs to read it." I've been told I'm sensitive, funny, insightful, stupid, an idiot, moronic, pedestrian, articulate, clever, caring, harsh, naive, pompous, likeable, rude, mean, polite, too fat — and too skinny.

However, the bottom line is I would not have been labelled as anything if not for your willingness to spend some time with me each week. I know you have a lot to do with too few hours in a day; yet here we are; you, me, and a few hundred words. For that, I'm honored, humbled — and extremely grateful. Short of a sincere "thank you," I am at a loss as to what to say, so much for winning a Pulitzer.

UNDERSTANDING WHAT DRIVES THE NEED FOR CHANGE

As much as I appreciate the Holidays, one has to admit it possess a downside: the relentless, unceasing, non-stop drone of promotions, commercials, and ads; loosely wrapped in pseudo-emotion by manipulative agencies pretending to appear as caring; with a primary objective being no more than inflating their coffers at our expense.

I do not consider all shopkeepers as greedy and soulless. Most are you and I, working their day-to-day, attempting to keep their heads above water. I also take no issue with profitability; we each must pay our bills. I am self-employed and therefore extremely aware of what it's like to stare at the ceiling all night concerned how to pay my vendors, keep the government satisfied; and still claim some folding money for my family.

But can we be honest? After 132 renditions of the "Night Before Christmas" re-written into unusual off-tone radio commercials, can we unite hand-in-hand and admit that it wears down the psyche?

Deepak Chopra, lecturer and author, stated in December, "We are spending money we don't have to buy things we don't need to impress people we don't like."

Ouch. That kind of hurts; but "why?"

Statements containing some inner truth are the only ones that wound us. As example, should someone tell you "you're a lousy golfer," and you've never walked a course, nor do you know a divot from a dogleg; you would take no offense, your emotional well-being remaining fully intact. Yet, should your child shout, "you're a horrible mother," that might inflict some pain. Although we know she is acting out, if we possess ANY insecurity about the subject — no matter no minute — and someone casts light upon it, we cannot help but flinch. Inner doubts multiply rapidly.

So as we again slog through the silly season of resolutions, it's time to take inner stock.

One cannot toss a week-old fruitcake three feet without hitting an advertisement proclaiming "flatter abs" or "30 pound weight loss." Every jolly, chubby, singing elf TV advertisement has been displaced with ads portraying an eye-poppingly gorgeous bikini-clad woman possessing a figure-not-found-in-nature, emerging from a swimming pool (in January, really??). As the water slithers from her tanned lean limbs, she pauses and proclaims, "With my new miracle ab-dissolver, I've lost 83 pounds and turned my life around — in the last thirty days. My children now behave. My husband can't keep his hands off me — and we even won the lottery." Standing by her side is masculine tanned, eye candy with a sculpted jaw, and a stomach so taunt one could cut diamonds on it. He beams lovingly at his wife, eyes twinkling, and in unison, staring directly into the lens, they ask, "What are YOU waiting for?"

Intuitively, logically, we know it's a set up. But it appeals to our inner sense of "wrongness" because we already feel bad about ourselves. In that emotional Achilles' heel, deliverance is at hand, in the form of an 800 number. Redemption lies in the phone operators who are standing by for the next 22 minutes; for only with their assistance (and $24.95 in shipping and handling) can we convert our ugly ducklingness to swans. Due to this primal knee-jerk reaction to be "fixed," there are millions of treadmills serving as no more than expensive coat hangers.

This column is not a thesis for stasis, rather a call to rational long-term thinking. Change or die is reality. However, change approached from a place of inner strength yield vastly improved, longer-lasting results. It's okay to be proud of who you are — while still on the road to getting better.

LUCKY NUMBERS

Numbers loom large in our lives. We commemorate birthdays and anniversaries in numbers of years. We monitor wealth in number of dollars. We even categorize our state of being via numbers: IQ, BMI, HDL.

Certain numbers are more popular than others. Take the number "3." We're conditioned to "think in 3s," which explains why we use expressions like "Top three reasons…" or "Three examples…" Angry parents rely on "3." My father, when upset, never said, "I'm going to count to four;" I'm guessing yours didn't either.

One is a "power number" too, so when I woke up New Year's day and noted the date, 1.1.11, I thought, "How cool!" Only nine times per century is every numeral in a date identical. My first "matched set" was 5.5.55 - but I was too young to fully appreciate it. Should I get a second chance in these next 100 years, I assure you there will be extreme gratitude.

However, 1.1.11 caused me to ponder, "Is there special significance from four "1"s? Might there be a cosmic sign in the only year that truly begins at the beginning? I'm not superstitious; but what about lucky numbers? What could "1.1.11" be trying to communicate?

In binary "1111" is "15." Maybe this year's providential number is 15? However, with the exception of the Fiesta Quinceañera, "15" doesn't show up much in our society.

So, I turned to numerology. In full disclosure, numerology is a topic about which I know zero (an unfortunate "power number). I could not tell my Soul Urge Number from my street address. But, I believe there is a lot of adding numerals together (or maybe there isn't; like I said I really know nothing about it). Either way, that's what I did. I added 1+5 from "15" to get "6" which seemed more probable than "15." After all, it's literally in the top ten of numbers. (Why don't we say "Top Nine" or "Top 11?" See… there we go again…)

Yet, if I'm adding, why not use the sum of all the ones? Wouldn't that make more sense? So, "4" must be the positive omen we need for the next 365 days.

Oy! Now I'm confused. We have three promising numbers: 15, 6, 4. Add those and the result is "25." Two+5=7. Seven could work; that feels right. But "7" is so commonplace and run of the mill; everybody and their brother uses "lucky 7."

Maybe I'm working this too hard. It's obvious. Staring me right in the kisser is the solution; it's a great big honkin' "ONE." And if we're looking at a new year as an opportunity to change, "1" squares perfectly with it. Most people do not achieve their goals (or "resolutions" if you insist) not because they're too small, but for the opposite reason: they make too many of them and they're ridiculously complicated. With great intention, but poor planning, they devise 46-step action plans, with options, timetables, flow-charts, and alternatives. Who has time to keep track of all that? The result? We get overwhelmed and intimidated. We feel bad and when that happens, we give up, feeling it's more trouble than it's worth, which is usually true. So, nothing happens. It's a horrible vicious cycle we repeat year after year.

To counter that, what's simpler than "1"?

If "1.1.11" is an omen, it's telling us "simplify." Pick ONE thing each day. Do it until completion. Repeat as necessary. After all, ONE goal here and ONE goal there done well can really add up to ONE happy life.

Toning Down the Language

There was a shooting tragedy in Tucson last week. I'm sure you're aware of it; you'd have to live in a hole to not to be.

At this writing, this horrific event does not seem motivated as much by politics (e.g. the Oklahoma Bombing) as it is by the fact that the shooter was mentally unstable, such as those at Columbine. (I'm sure this is small comfort to the families of the victims.) Nonetheless, finger-pointing began per schedule. Blame will be assessed, and as with a New Year's resolution, promises will be made. For a brief moment, our awareness will be heightened and actions might be taken. Unfortunately, also like those resolutions, these commitments will be abandoned in short order.

I am loath to wish for the "good old days." First of all, I don't believe that the times when polio existed, racism was accepted, and children would "drop and cover" to practice for nuclear attacks; were "good old days." Secondly, lamenting what has already passed is useless. Even if the past was as pristine and idyllic as some would like to remember, it is indeed just that: past. That said, during those bygone days our elected representatives might have been at odds with each other on the congressional floor, yet they retained a sense of civility, even friendship, when day was done. This has, so it appears, been lost of late as both sides have become armed camps; shaking out positions, with nary a thought of middle ground.

Therefore, one positive outcome arising from this tragedy (if "positive" can be the label applied to anything that comes of it) is the heightened scrutiny on the tone of the political discourse during this fractious era. Only time will tell if it was a partial cause in the shooter's break with humanity; but it cannot be a bad thing to examine. The heat has been turned up on the uncivil rhetoric espoused by many in the public spotlight. They are apparently feeling that heat because the common reply is "We have to tone it down on both sides." Here is where I have an unlikely concern: As long as the meme is "both sides are responsible," neither side will take action. Whenever we can point fingers at someone else, even if others are pointing at us, we have an "out," an escape, a way to avoid the responsibility we hold.

I am not simply speaking of hate-speech nor of calls to incite violence, this concept also applies to a much more basic level of personal responsibility and change. Until we accept that the "we" must "tone it down;" "we" must change (on whatever level that is applicable), there is always a scapegoat and a way out. Being human; we are quite likely to take it.

If change is truly our goal - whether it is our political discourse or our personal lives - we must understand that the only thing we can change is "us." And the only part of "us" over which I have control is "me."

You and I make up the "we." I will watch more closely what I say, both to you and to myself. I hope you will do the same, but I have very little control over that; for the only part of this green planet I do control is the few square feet in which I exist. At least I can make that a better place for all who come in contact with it.

FAREWELL TO AN OLD FRIEND

When she was a kitten, we were constantly cleaning up remnants of paper. We'd leave the house and return to scraps of napkins scattered about the kitchen, or the roll of toilet paper splayed from bathroom to living room. Paper products lived in fear if KC Whittinger Long-stockings Junior was nearby.

I'll place squarely the blame on my sons who chose her moniker (which might not be accurate but I can do that because they don't live here and won't be able to read this). "KC" was short for "Kitty Cat" (not very imaginative, I know). I don't know the derivation of the rest of her handle but it didn't matter; we referred to her simply as "KC" or "Case-ers."

I specifically chose KC because she was the most talkative cat in the litter and I wanted company. As they say, "Be careful what you wish for…" Not only did she communicate, she did it — shall we say — "with enthusiasm." She had a habit of waiting stealthily in the early morning darkness in the kitchen. The first human to enter would be "greeted" with an enormous, howling ululation. Never sure whether it was "Good Morning," or "What the heck took you so long to fill my bowl?," what I can assure you is that after being welcomed as such, there was no longer a need to use coffee to start your heart.

As a kitten, she adamantly refused to drink water inside the house. We placed bowls strategically throughout the rooms; a guest entering our home for the first time and seeing the water filled containers scattered hither and yon would assume we had the leakiest roof in the neighborhood. It was of no consequence; she refused to drink from them. When thirst took hold, she would sit patiently by the back door until we conceded to her wishes. Then she'd sway and saunter on to the deck and lap only from the bowl outside. It was a ritual we referred to as "Water in the Wild."

She rumbled constantly, purring simply if you looked at her, louder if you touched her. Of course she purred when she ate (how do they do that?), purred when she cleaned, and purred when she drank. She would purr, well, just because she could.

Since we kept the door to the downstairs closed at night, she trained my younger son to wake up at any hour, open it, and sit drearily by her side in the event of her need for a midnight snack. He would complain about it; yet repeat the ritual whenever KC deemed it necessary. My wife and I found it funny, looking at them as an old married couple who seem to irritate each other to no end, but in reality, actually love each other deeply.

Even though her attitude never changed, she succumbed to the tolls of aging and slowed in her last few years. Due to a metabolism problem, she lost a great deal of weight; her fur became ragged, she moved more cautiously, and would sleep almost continually. Since her teeth were failing, I took her to the vet last week for a routine procedure that would help her eat with less pain, causing her to gain some weight, and hopefully feel better. It didn't work out that way.

She never came home.

It's funny how we can bond so closely to something that weighs less than a sack of potatoes. I know some day we shall purr again, but right now, it's time to heal.

Five things you can do to be happier and more successful starting NOW

Improving oneself is not difficult. It might be uncomfortable. It might be slow; but difficult? Not so much. Figure out what you want to change; figure out a way to do it, move in that direction, correct as necessary.

So why don't most people change? The unadorned answer is we make it too complicated. The simpler the plan, the more likely we will accomplish it. To that end, here is a straightforward Five-Step Plan to move forward immediately.

1) Write it down

There's nothing magic to this, but once done, it makes it "real." It also helps if we don't just write down what we want but why we want it. Emotions drive action. Logic directs it. As example, "I will lose weight to lower my blood pressure," is not as effective as "I will lose weight to feel better." As they say in sales, "We buy what we want, not necessarily what we need." We need to "sell" ourselves on why we want it more than why we should do it.

2) Make it Small

Small steps done regularly generate better results than large steps done intermittently. In other words, it's better to get out a walk a block - and really do it - than to swear you're going to run a mile and plant yourself on the couch. We have to "squeeze" new activities into an already crowded life so the less we have to rearrange, the more likely we'll be consistent. Ten or 15-minutes with consistency is better than "an occasional hour."

3) Do Something Every Day

No matter how small the step, do SOMETHING each day, even if it's simply refining what we wrote. Maintaining top-of-mind awareness retrains our thoughts to focus differently. That alone causes us to notice previously unseen opportunities.

Of course, there are days when "life happens" and we cannot move forward, which can bring out our critical inner perfectionists and we are inclined to think, "As long as I blew it, I might as well really blow it. I'll start again tomorrow." This leads to undoing our progress. It's important to remember everyone stumbles; progress is two steps forward and one step backwards.

4) Get Support

There are things we do well and there are things we want to do well. Making life-changes falls in the latter category, not the former. After all, if we were accomplished at our goals, we would have already achieved them. Building a network of support can guide and direct us when we feel lost, and applaud us when we aren't. There is always more power in a group than in a single person (for better or worse).

One other benefit to group support is it "shuts the back door." Too often, we don't tell people our goals because if do, we have to actually change. Well, short of the fact that you can change your mind, announcing our plans does make us more committed to achieving them. Keeping them "quiet" allows us to back down quicker, which prompts the question, "Am I really committed to this?" (a discussion left for another column)

5) Reward Yourself Often

Change is as much emotional as it is physical. Holding off the goodies from our "inner kid," makes us feel like we've got one more chore in an already tedious life. We get resentful and quit. If however, we can make it more fun, we're more inclined to keep at it Life is short, enjoy it - and remind yourself more often of the pleasures.

BEING GRATEFUL FOR A BIKE ACCIDENT

With clear skies and a light breeze, it was weather made for a leisurely bicycle commute. I peddled merrily, admiring the scenery, breathing deep the cool air, grateful for being alive. All was as it should be; at least until the gremlins got me.

It began with a random thought, "Did you close the garage door?"

Understand, I have never left the garage open when I've left my house so there's no reason to assume I had done anything but that. Yet, the more I tried to turn down the noise, the louder it became. With every crank of the pedals, the more I worried. Deciding I was ruining a perfectly good ride, I opted to return home and confirm the house was indeed secure.

To turn around, I pulled into a driveway but due to its narrow width, I couldn't complete the action. I tried to put my feet down but due to the slope of the driveway, combined with my less-than-towering height, I couldn't reach the ground and lost balance. Upon realizing gravity was going to win this battle, I stretched out my arms to cushion the blow, landing with a severe THUD on the curb next to a garbage can. My right hand took the brunt of the impact; shortly before my jaw bounced against the concrete and my ribs smashed against the tubular frame of the bike, leaving me in a tangle on the street.

As cars passed, I wondered if anyone would stop, or did they consider a middle-age guy laying in the sewer some sort of performance art or misplaced garbage?

"Look honey, isn't that a man sprawled in the gutter?"

"By Jove, I think you're right!"

"Do you think we should see if he's okay?"

"Why should we? It looks like the people in that house tried to throw him away, but missed the can. We don't have time to pick up other people's trash. However, you'd think they'd have more pride in the appearance of their property, don't you?"

With a collective "Harrumph," and noses turned skyward, they would drive on. Whether or not that was the conversation, no one stopped.

I assessed the damage. My jaw and hand were already throbbing but I was obviously conscious. I could — with much pain — move my fingers and my mouth. My chest ached; yet I could breathe. The bike was fine; my mirror and light were askew; but simple to fix.

With no small amount of effort, I pulled myself to vertical; considered my options, and came to the thankful realization "on the grand scale of things," it could have been worse. I was startled I at how grateful I was.

Therein lies the lesson. Most of the time, "it could be worse" and someday "it will be worse." But not right NOW — and that's where I live, right now. I'm no Pollyanna; I understand "stuff happens," yet I was able to continue on with my plans and make it home just fine (albeit more slowly). There are people whose daily experiences are far worse than most of what happens to me in an entire lifetime. When I put it into that perspective, I am grateful. When I dramatically lament, "woe is me," it does feel worse.

As a dear friend reminded me, "When everything seems crazy, remember to breathe" (even if my ribs hurt).

Oh yes, I had locked the garage door.

February Resolutions

We're six weeks into the year; so, how are those New Year's resolutions workin' for ya?

If they're now broken shards lying along the highway shoulder several miles in the rear view mirror, fret not, you stand not alone. According to surveys, as many as 80 percent of people give up their vast and glorious seemed-like-a-good-idea-at-the-time plans by the tail end of January; more alarming is as many as 90 percent are never brought to fruition. What might the foremost reasons for not accomplishing them be? About 40 percent of respondents say they didn't have enough time (read that "not a high enough priority") and about one-third say they weren't even committed to doing them in first place. Basically, they set them to get someone off their back. Yep, nothing says "motivation to change" like a heaping, steaming pile of guilt.

Personally, I think the "New Year's Resolution" is a manufactured event; akin to holidays we didn't know existed until we went into the greeting card shop. We respond to public pressure, and since "everyone's doing it," we don't want to pay the social price for not going along; hence we make promises we never intend to keep.

Nothing's wrong with January 1; I mean why not, it's as good date as any. But change drives its own train and you better get on board when it's time or you'll be left at the station. If your marriage is monotonous and unsatisfying on April 7, you might be single in seven months. Having trouble seeing your belt buckle without looking in the mirror? Why wait? After all, your belly's not going to shrink by itself, is it? Or, if you get up most mornings with an "ain't-life-a-drag hangover," it might seem the perfect date for a decision is the one that's staring you in the face on the calendar.

I don't mean to be snarky but in the interest of trying to make a point, the perfect date for change is, well, today. If you re-read this tomorrow, that works also. Yet, per my previous comments, most of us like to feel we're not alone in our quest; so ever the helper, by the power vested in me (which admittedly isn't much), I proclaim February 15 as the first annual "This Time I Mean It Day." (Please insert your own trumpets.) I am attempting to get as many people as possible to recommit to objectives delayed — and equally as important, to celebrate those things we have accomplished already, while supporting others as they reach upward also.

It might appear out of the norm to discuss resolutions when red roses, heart-adorned boxer shorts, and enough chocolate to give us a yearlong cocoa high surround us; but there's method to my madness. The date was specifically chosen to coincide with the holiday most dedicated to commitment: Valentine's Day.

When we care about someone and we value the relationship, we take those extra moments to engage in those additional activities that ease their burdens, lighten their load, and lift them up. If we care about ourselves, it seems we need no less. After all, if we don't take care of us, who will take care of everyone we take care of? (I know; that sentence is horribly constructed but you get the point.)

So, onward self-improving soldiers, carpe diem! Make a commitment. Take a step. Share it with a friend. Don't worry about joining late; we'll still be marching on February 16th, June 17th, or any day thereafter. The road never ends.

WHAT REALLY MATTERS IS USUALLY RIGHT IN FRONT OF US

 ⌒

Imagine what life would be like if we each lived exactly 100 years — to the day. From the moment of birth, barring accidents, you knew the exact minute of your death. One some levels it could be reassuring; however, as the calendar years passed, it might get a little freaky. There would be no doubt about how much time was left on your clock.

With that as the backdrop, pretend you are now 99 years and 364 days old, it's your last day on the planet. You have all the knowledge you can possibly acquire. Whatever you have attempted is considered complete. Your trials, tribulations, and triumphs have left their marks. Lessons have been learned. Knowledge has been acquired. Whatever else you had planned will remain unaccomplished. There is nothing left to do but look back and analyze the story of your life.

Your time has come.

Using that scenario, suppose you could "send a message" back to the real-life YOU of today, the person reading these words this very minute. You would say, "In your remaining years, always remember and stay focused on what rally matters," and you would list those top priorities so present-day you wouldn't reach the end of life filled with regrets for being out of alignment.

In an exercise to establish priorities, I have conducted an activity like this with audiences of all shapes and stripes, estimating the total number of people who have done this with me to be several thousand, maybe more. Some have shared their answers; it is not a surprise that almost all are priorities such as: take care of my family, have faith, be healthy, treat others well, smile often, love deeply, or improve my community. I am reassured that I can count on the fingers of one hand when someone shared a dream like "bright red sports car" or "a hot babe."

I find this wonderfully reassuring because I interpret these hopeful results as meaning that we, as a people, do seem to have a good direction. I think what happens is we get so mired in the day-to-day muck, we forget the big picture. We have our nose so close to the grindstone and our back so bent with our labors, that instead of focusing on what matters, all we get are sore lats and a flattened proboscis.

How often do we not even notice something wonderful that's right in front of us? As example, for Valentine's Day, my wonderful wife arose first and hung a bright red, shiny banner proclaiming, "I love you forever" at the entrance to our living room. Shortly thereafter, oblivious, I staggered out of bed and wandered into the living room, not noticing it, even as it almost brushed my head. I did observe something that needed to be put in the kitchen so I dutifully picked it up and left the room; still unobservant. I poured a cup of coffee and returned to the living room. I am embarrassed that I had still not noticed the banner.

My wife, upstairs, calls out, "Happy Valentines Day Honey," assuming of course, that with three trips to the living room, I must have seen her handiwork.

I replied, "You too honey."

She says, "What did you think?"

"About what?" I call back.

She says, "You didn't even see it?"

"See what?"

How many things of beauty do we miss each day, because we forget to look at what really matters? I am keeping my eyes more open today.

The Common Sense Diet

"Lose 20 pounds in one week! No dieting! No exercise! No lifestyle change!"

I will admit that I've been sucked in by such snake oil pitches and pie-in-the-sky promises ever since I was first embarrassed by having to shop in the "husky" section of the boys' clothing department. Yet, decades later, such 127-point screaming headline proclamations remain as common fare across the back pages of tabloids; or enthusiastically, breathlessly broadcast on slick, highly produced infomercials featuring questionable "experts" interviewing "real people" experiencing "actual results."

When we can turn down the magical thinking long enough to strap on our adult brain thinking caps, we know that losing weight is not rocket science; it's a simple premise; keep your mouth shut longer and your feet moving further and you'll end up at your correct weight. The bottom line is quite simply "calories in versus calories out." Period; end of story; mystery over. Spend more than you take in and — voila! — a new skinny you.

Should you need validation of this fact, the New England Journal of Medicine published a report a while ago, that proved that as long as a diet reduced one's caloric intake, the result was weight loss — regardless of the diet's make up of fat, protein, or carbohydrate. They asked 811 overweight and obese adults to try one of four different low-fat, high fiber diets. Activity was encouraged, and participants could receive group and individual support to keep them motivated. What they discovered was that craving, fullness, hunger, and diet satisfaction were similar across all four diets; and that all participants lost weight and reduced their waistlines — irrespective of the type of diet they followed.

Dr. Yoni Freedhoff, medical director of the Bariatric Medical Institute in Ottawa, says the study's results are good news for those who hate dieting, mentioning that the key to success is to find something you like so you will stick to it for the necessary period required to obtain your goal. "If (people) are trying to adhere to a diet they don't like, it's not going to work long term. If you don't like it now, you won't like it two years down the road. So whatever you are doing, if you don't like it, try something else."

Of course, common sense must prevail; not all calories are created equal and the real objective is good health, not simply a number on a scale. As illustration, let's assume your body needs about 1500 calories a day to maintain its weight. You decide you want to lose a pound a week, requiring you to shed approximately 500 calories a day. To do this, you switch to the "all beer diet." "Drink only beer and lose weight!" the promoters proclaim. At about 125 calories per serving, that equates to eight servings a day and nothing else.

Question: Would you lose weight?

Answer: Sure, it's calories in versus calories out.

Question two: Would you be healthy?

Answer: Not a chance. You might be skinny, but you'd be a wreck.

I'd love to be the one to unveil a new magical solution to weight loss; on that requires neither changes nor adjustments. I'd also like to be able to flap my arms and fly. Neither is going to happen. However, if I flap often enough, I could burn off a few calories; drop a few pounds, and even firm up that wiggly part under my arms.

"COMBO-PILLING" FOR WEIGHT LOSS, A BAD IDEA

While watching the news this morning, I was alerted to the practice of "combo-pilling," taking supposedly unrelated medications together to produce more powerful results toward a desired outcome. Combo-pilling diet drugs went mainstream in the 1980s, with the pairing of phentermine and fenfluramine (later known as "fen-phen"). This pairing, as well as a commercial related version, was heralded as the first effective weight loss drug treatment. Later, when it was discovered that the commercial drug was associated with potentially fatal pulmonary hypertension and heart-valve problems, it was withdrawn from the market and the manufacturer was sued to the tune of more than ten billion dollars.

Combo-pilling remains, in part because single diet drugs have not yielded the results many seek. After sibutramine (Meridia) was removed from market late last year, the only FDA-approved drug for treating obesity for more than a few weeks is orlistat. However, if dieters eat fat-heavy meals, the results are some less-than-pleasant side effects (oily stains on one's underwear, being one).

So combo-pilling continues.

Of late, the blend of Topomax, an anticonvulsant approved for the treatment of epilepsy and migraines; and phentermine, the above referenced appetite suppressant, are making their way into the collective dieters' consciousness. It appears that Topomax effectively "shuts off" the desire to eat. When combined with phentermine, the results can be downright staggering. I monitored some on-line discussion groups and found it not uncommon for participants to claim weight losses of four or five pounds a week for extended periods. (A healthy sustainable weight loss is considered to be one to two pounds per week.)

Using medicine for what it is not intended is called "off-label" use. Although no official data exist as to the extent of this practice, a March 2009 study published in Obesity found that 65 percent of weight specialists belonging to the American Society of Bariatric Physicians who responded to a survey do indeed prescribe "off-label" combinations. The practice is legal; in fact, according to a 2006 analysis in the Archives of Internal Medicine, approximately 20 percent of common adult drugs are prescribed as such. (Since the drug is approved and on the market, physicians may use it as they see fit.)

While some doctors are unconcerned, many are raising red flags, pointing out that these medical "cocktails" might be taken for years, causing long-term adverse interactions and unexpected side effects. Since the FDA is not monitoring such usage, authorities might never find out about such problems; and even if they do, it could lead to catastrophic results for those experimenting with untested combinations.

Referencing the aforementioned Internet discussions, the danger seems to be of little concern to some who insist on doing "whatever it takes" to achieve their correct weight; consequences be damned. Said one post, "I started … one week ago and I've lost eight pounds already. I agree with the post above that this may not be 'healthy' weight loss, but being overweight isn't healthy either. If this gets me to a healthy weight, then so be it." Alarming, isn't it?

Of greater concern to me is not the threat of obesity, but that being overweight is considered such a stigma and so abhorrent that some would literally risk life and limb to drop pounds. If it is indeed so vital to lose the weight, wouldn't it seem like it might be important enough to rearrange one's life to eat a less and walk a little more? It's a slower process, yes; but the worst side effects in that situation are a growling belly and sore feet.

A REMINDER OF WHAT REALLY MATTERS

It seems like merely days ago the public dialogue bounced between the skyrocketing price of groceries and gasoline; the rising up of working people in the mid east — as well as our own mid west; and the ramblings of a seemingly unstable, implausibly garrulous celebrity whose veins course with "dragon's blood." It seems like just days ago because, well, it was.

Time zips by without delay and such topics are soooooo last week. In point of fact, nothing has changed except our attention. One still needs to refinance his house to purchase groceries (if he can find a willing bank); riots and unrest in northern Africa continue; and that particular celebrity — well, he just won't shut up, will he?

Yet, we have been radically refocused.

My wife woke me last Friday with alarm in her voice, "There was a huge quake in Japan. It's triggered a tsunami warning here." As it turned out, we were spared; however, when I flipped on the television to find out what evacuation might entail, I — probably like you — witnessed the horrific, gut-wrenching images of a "first-world country" laid low by a one-two gut punch of earthquake and its resultant tsunami; the strength of which not only literally moved Japan, but shifted the Earth's axis, and even altered time.

How can mere mortals come to terms with the concept of such seemingly unlimited power? It is indeed reminder that we reside on Mother Earth at her pleasure; a privilege she may revoke at any time with nothing greater than a flick of her authority. It is humbling to realize how inconsequential are we in relationship to the planet on which we exist.

Do not misconstrue my statement as, "We are insignificant." Quite the contrary, we are awesome creatures with immeasurable capabilities, blessed with brilliance, and gifted with limitless grace and goodness. It's just that — once in a while — we get lost. We forget. We bind ourselves into knots about events and activities that mean — on the grand scale of things — virtually nothing.

I whine about being delayed by excess red lights when I'm rushing to an appointment. I complain to the clerk about the cost of fruit, as if she does not have to deal with it for her own household budget. I boil with rage when I reflect on the contractor who never correctly fixed our leaky roof. Each of us has our "ain't-life-awful list," which we are so quick to pull out and share whenever needed (and usually when not).

To put it in perspective, my car is a "beater," but it's also not crushed under the rubble of what was my house. I am able to go where I want, when I want, while driving on (mostly-intact) roads. Food might be pricey, but I am not in an endless queue hoping for a relief truck, donned in a mask as a thin barrier against disease and an expanding nuclear disaster. Yes, my roof really leaks; no, it shouldn't. It's damn frustrating. But, I am not sleeping in a tent of bed sheets in freezing temperatures neither. Until the leak is repaired, all I need to is place a bucket on the floor and sidestep the wet place.

As they say, "There but for the Grace of God goes any of us." We survive. We are mostly comfortable. For those, be grateful. Yet, with gratitude comes responsibility. We must provide what we can to those who are enduring so much. It could be us, and we would hope for no less.

"When combined with a healthy diet..."

Until moments ago, I was unaware of the term, "to throw a wobbly."

Looking for a more colorful way to declare, "I am annoyed," I stumbled upon the expression at a website devoted entirely to idioms and their etymology. (Fellow word geeks unite! Our time has arrived!)

Sure, I guess I could have simply said, "I am annoyed." There's nothing wrong with that. It's clear, simple, to the point. However, fashioning myself as crafts person of the language arts, I forever seek out-of-the-ordinary turns of a phrase to spice up how I communicate, the intent being to make it more vivid and engaging. Not being much of a cook, I presume it's in the same manner as a chef would feel if confined to white salt and black pepper. Sure, they'll do the job; but where's the fun?

Should you — like me — have been in the dark about "throwing a wobbly;" let me explain. Turns out, it's not a good substitution for "annoyed." Rather, it appears to be of British or Australian derivation, coined from the adjective "wobbled" which meant someone was "off center." So, "throwing a wobbly" can best be described as a petulant rant; somewhat akin to "throwing a hissy fit." It is however not as severe as "going ballistic." Now, don't we feel smart?

Alas, it's still not the correct usage for what I want so it's back to being annoyed; or maybe cranky. I don't know; can one be both? Sure, why not?

Hmmm, I seem to have digressed. The bigger issue is, "What prompted said (poorly described) uncomfortable emotional state?" I shall explain.

Today's email heralded an e-solicitation from an unheard of someone looking to introduce me to a nutritional protein shake that "can be used as a meal replacement for weight loss and better health." Not interested in hawking the product, but apparently driven by a more pressing desire to procrastinate on more urgent deadlines, I opted to follow the web link. The page materialized with imagery of beautiful bodies, healthy meals, thick chocolate shakes, and, of course, a prominent "Order Now" button.

According to the text, if I drink just one shake a day "and follow a healthy diet and exercise plan," I will "lose weight, lower my cholesterol, shed inches, and improve digestion." Curiosity now engaged, I searched the Internet for dietary aids, and realized virtually every site had a similar disclaimer: "…when combined with a healthy diet and exercise plan…" It might not have been prominent (usually wasn't); but there it was, plain as day; just like the six-pack abs on the smiling male model.

See, here's the thing. Should I weigh too much, and should I then choose to "follow a healthy diet and exercise regularly," I will have no choice but to "lose weight, lower my cholesterol, shed inches, and improve digestion." It has nothing to do with powders, pills, or potions. Moreover, I can take the money saved to purchase new clothing to better adorn my now-healthier, happier body.

It's not that such products are all without value; if they help you stay on track, and they're healthy, and you can afford them, well, as they say, "You go girl!" Yet, it's vital to remember there is no "magic shake" substitute for behavior change. Until one is willing to make the mental shift from "it's about what I eat" to "it's about how I live," she will continue to be frustrated enough with the results to throw a wobbly.

HANDLING STRESS

How do I stress thee? Let me count the ways.
I am stressed to the depth and breadth and height
That gas prices can reach, seemingly out of sight
From the ends of my soul to the lines on my face.

I am anxious of wars, and disasters aplenty
Of leaders who don't and anger abounding,
Anxiety, frustration, worries, throughout life,
I have stressors galore; I need some relief.

…with sincere apologies to Elizabeth Barrett Browning

Have you noticed that life seems a bit catawampus lately? Watching the news can launch a full-fledged panic attack. Granted, there is an off switch for your electronics, but you cannot unplug the outlandish price of groceries, $4 a gallon gasoline, or job furloughs. Many of us may be suffering post traumatic stress disorder, complicated by the fact that it's not yet "post," it's "current," with no let-up in sight.

I playfully refer to this column as a "a cross between Attitude 101, therapy, and a southern revival." I try to add some insights into the human condition with a sincere interest in lightening its load. Although helpful, I attempt to make these 600 words upbeat and light as often as possible.

Alas, I also happen to be human and therefore succumb to the same moods as anyone else. Of late, I have been gloomier than is my norm. Even though therapists would remind, "there is no such thing as a negative feeling," I insist on shaking off this type of mood as quickly as possible. It might be "normal," yet I still do not want to marinate in it. The problem was it was particularly sticky and my usual tools were ineffective, so hi-ho, hi-ho, it's off to research I go.

I discovered that stress is the body's reaction to change, any change; the more significant or unexpected, the more the stress. Lots of change ("stressors") becomes lots of stress. To reduce it, we can try to restore some balance or normalcy by:

- Accepting the reality of how we feel. We are emotional beings; our feelings are every bit as real an aspect of us as are our arms or legs. Denying them will not make them vanish. Worse, not only can it delay resolution (can you say "denial?"), but it can also damage our health, which leads to the next tip…

- Move. We are also physical beings. Our bodies react to those feelings and thoughts. If we feel unable to change them, we sure as heck can change the position of our bodies. It can be as simple as taking a walk or even standing instead of sitting; anything that's out of the usual. Change your position; you will change your mood.

- Reach out. Of course, we are also social, which explains why we build communities and relationships. It's who we are at our core. Talk to someone. Remember, even powerful people have needs. Besides, when you share, you almost immediately feel better.

- Express gratitude. This might seem odd; after all, it appears that there's very little for which to give thanks. Yet, happier people (i.e. less stressed) also tend to be more thankful. It's a chicken and egg thing; which comes first? Find something — anything — for which to be grateful. Focus on it for a moment. (Please pass it on. We can all use the reminder.)

We're going to be here for a while. We can object to it — and by golly, I'm sure we will — but we also need to do something about it. Taking care of each other can't hurt, even when things improve.

"UM, WHAT WERE WE TALKING ABOUT?"

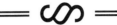

Pop quiz! What did they call "multitasking" in the eighties?

Answer: "lack of focus."

I don't mean to sound like an old fuddy-duddy (of course, using the term "fuddy-duddy" does tend to portray me as such), but like it or not, I am officially of a "certain age." More times than I care to admit, I have strutted with strong intention into the kitchen, and upon arrival, completely blanked as to why I was there. Or, finding myself looking for an item in the closet, I will be briefly distracted, and forget what I was looking for. I have, embarrassingly enough, "lost" my keys on the way to the door on more than one occasion.

My wife and I have entire conversations without ever using proper nouns.

"Hi Honey, I saw that guy today."

"Which guy?"

"You know, the man who did the thing around the house last summer."

"Oh, with the stuff and that equipment?"

"No, the other one. He worked on the what-do-you-call-it with those tools. You know, over by that place..."

"Oh, him! With all that oily gear?"

"Yeah, him."

"Why didn't you just say so?"

We're not trying to be secretive; it's simply that the words don't form as quickly as we need so, undeterred, we press on in the language of "pronouncia." (What's bizarre is we actually understand each other.)

Distractions are prominent in my work, which causes me to regularly bounce from one task to another. As illustration, the vast majority of my time is in front of a computer monitor. I might be — as I am now — writing a column. Whilst engaged in said project, my email program beeps, alerting me to a new message. Like a bright shiny object on a string in front of a cat, I immediately shift gears to examine it. The sender included a link; now I find myself online, searching for a new book. Not remembering the title I wanted, I go to our bookcase for inspiration. There I notice an accumulation of dust, requiring me to retrieve the vacuum cleaner. This routes me through the kitchen and it dawns on me that I must eat. Since I am forever dieting, I track everything I consume, so I return to the computer to do so and remember that today is "bill-paying" day. To get organized for the endeavor, I rearrange my file cabinet— until I recall that I was on deadline. I return to the original mission, having accomplished none of my interim goals and now desperately behind schedule. Oy vey!

So it comes as no surprise that a report this week finds older people have less of an ability to multi-task, possibly because they can't refocus as well after getting interrupted. Dr. Adam Gazzaley, the study's co-author, explains, "Older adults pay too much attention to the irrelevant information." The problem is they (we?) have "trouble switching back" to the issue at hand and disengaging from the interruption.

The difficulty with multitasking is that we can't really focus on multiple assignments all at once, said Russell A. Poldrack, a psychology professor in Texas. "We are almost always switching back and forth between the different tasks, and there is a cost to this switching, which is why people are nearly always worse when they try to multi-task compared to focusing on single tasks." The solution, according to Mr. Poldrack is — if you absolutely have to multi-task — "improve general brain health, and the best way that we know [to do that] is aerobic exercise."

I hope I can remember that.

The problem with deprivation diets

If deprivation was a successful weight loss strategy, obesity would be obliterated.

At first blush, sacrificing one's favorites appears like it would blast away those extra pounds, and it does —but only temporarily. Long-term, it's unnatural and ineffective.

Oh, sure, we can sacrifice our pet foods for brief periods. However, let's face it, as the joke goes, seven days of bland makes one weak. Without variety, we get bored. Take away our special beloved "fun foods" and we give up, sometimes in horrifying ways.

As example, I decide to implement a new "healthy me lifestyle change," a complete makeover of my insalubrious habits. My wife, ever the obliging supportive spouse; agrees to assist, so we commence a routine evening stroll. The weather is agreeable, walking burns calories, and the time allows us to re-connect after hectic workdays.

Along the route lies a small pizzeria. I am wise in the ways of weight loss and I know from unfortunate past experience, that the blend of salt, several varieties of cheese, as well as toasted doughy goodness, makes it problematic for me to lose weight. Therefore, I have sworn an oath of "pizza abstinence" until the scale reflects 15 fewer pounds. I am proud to announce that so far, all is going well. I've been "pizza-free" for well over three hours.

Fate however can be a cruel mistress and the gentle breeze this evening brings upon it a warm cheesy waft of mozzarella and garlic. As

Ulysses being lured by the Sirens, my wife grabs tighter my hand, the rope attempting to bind me to the mast. Unhappily, she is not composed of wood and twine and I tear loose, hot footing frenziedly into the eatery, no longer able to manage my impulse.

That's when things got fuzzy.

Although I do not recall the incident after that moment, I am informed by my lawyer that the SWAT team pulled me from atop the front, shaking a terrified 19-year-old clerk by the lapels, flop-sweat streaming from my brow, spaghetti sauce dripping from my lips, while shrieking "Extra cheese, more pepperoni, and three pounds of garlic sticks — and no one gets hurt!"

Okay, I exaggerated (my demand was only two pounds of garlic sticks) but many a well-intentioned dieter has been kicked to the curb by an unexpected overwhelming urge for verboten foodstuffs.

The reality is that over-eating is an addiction; it might be "small-A-addiction," but in many cases, it can be as debilitating as drugs or alcohol (and the societal cost is far greater). The difference is that with other addictions, one can go cold turkey. It might not be easy and one might need the support of others. Yet, a line in the sand can be drawn and never again crossed.

Food is obviously different. We need to learn to control our intake and to get away from the black/white, good/bad, on/off diet mentality. Thin people eat pizza. They eat chocolate too. Pay attention and you'll even observe folks with a healthy waistline engaging in a bag of tortilla chips or a large scoop of ice cream. The reason they're thin — and some of us are not — is that they don't freak out about what they eat. Should they overindulge, they adjust by eating less or exercising more. For them, it's habit. For the rest of us, it takes some thought, but anything of value usually does.

BUILDING SUPPORTIVE RELATIONSHIPS

In the end, we are remembered via the relationships we leave behind.

I stand five-eight, no one's depiction of "towering giant." Someone of my stature is supposed to tip the scales at no more than 165 pounds. When I was 39 years old, I weighed 250. More frightening was that at such an early age, I experienced chest pains with regularity. As a father for two young sons, I was a ghost. My career was in free fall; my 12-year marriage was in tatters. (When your marriage counsel or suggests divorce lawyers, the odds for regaining your long-lost marital bliss are slim.)

Change is born of fear, force, or pain. No one wakes up one fine day and says, "Wow! I really love my life; how am I going to change it?" Rather, unhappy, dissatisfied, and overwhelmed, we resolve to do virtually anything to alter our circumstances; anywhere is better than here.

For me, that conclusion came late one night, sitting alone yet again, pondering sorrowfully the source of my life's despair. Out of that sadness came the painful realization that the common bond among all my troubles was ME. It was ME who relinquished the reins of my life,it was ME who helped build a dysfunctional marriage, and it was ME who chose to stuff myself, medicating the hurt by eating instead of fixing it. Therefore, if anyone was going to transform my life, it too must be ME.

On stressful days, instead of eating, I started walked. I saw a therapist and I attended weight loss meetings. With such support, I learned to focus on what was triggering the urge to eat and avoid it, rather than lamenting the unhealthful decision when it was a fait de compli. Reacting differently created calm and peace, which in turn lowered the desire to "medicate," therefore causing weight loss and its resultant health and happiness.

My wife, noticing my enhanced outlook (and shrinking waistline) probed, "You're planning on leaving me, aren't you?"

I replied — honestly, "No. My plan is to become healthy. My sincere hope is you'll come with me — but I am going either way."

In the end, she opted not to.

When we alter our lives, step one is a conscious decision to do so. That's obvious. In our newfound zeal, what is less apparent is that the choices we make not only affect us, but all with whom we interact; children, co-workers, spouses, partners, and friends; to name a few. Equally true is that their timetables and needs might be dissimilar from our own; and they might not necessarily be ready, willing, or desirous of pursuing that same objective. Some will choose to support us. Others will slow our progress, while still others will leave us.

The sometimes-painful adjustments we make to achieve our true potential are not excuses to avoid doing what must be done. Yet they remind us that being healthy also means being aware of the impact our decisions have on those we care about. It is a sad reality that relationships come — and sometimes they do go. The better ones remain for long periods while others of less consequence exist so briefly, we don't even remember we had them.

As I told my children, "Compassion always; but don't be confused, the price of giving up your dreams is higher than the cost of letting go of painful relationships. That said, do what you can to repair them before you let them go. Other people are involved."

THE FANTASY OF
PERFECTIONISM

I am a perfect-o-holic.

Sure, I know it's folly; yet I can picture that magical happy place where all goes according to plan and everything works out as I imagined. I have a plan.

Today, I become the pinnacle of modern workplace efficiency. Without exception, every single solitary item on my to-do list will be accomplished — even those lingering on the pad since '07. Phone calls will be returned in a timely, upbeat, eager manner, complete with all the necessary and required information at hand. Today, every goal will be exceeded; every dead lines hall be beat. Should I spot a customer, client, co-worker, or vendor, I shall stretch out a warm enthusiastic hand in friendship, greeting her with passion, warmth, and energy; developing the ultimate positive reputation. Today, all reports will be finished on time and with precision. Today, the five-year backlog of filing shall be ended. Facebook farm games, really cute cat videos on You Tube, and forwarded emails with titles like "LOL! OMG! You've got to see this!" shall not deter me from my mission. I am a rock. (I shall be so effectual that I will have even had enough spare time to properly arrange my computer's desktop icons in perfect order. After all, I owe it to myself to have some fun.)

Moreover, I will not ignore my most important relationship. Mark this date; for it is when I became the perfect spouse. Should my loving wife require assistance, no matter what else I am doing, I shall immediately — sans attitude, of course — cease all other pursuits, and lavish upon her all the attention she so richly deserves. As illustration of how central is our shared life, I will make time to clean the bathroom, prepare dinner, wash the dishes, pay the bills, and even massage her aching feet, expecting nothing in return. Today, I am the perfect husband.

To achieve these lofty goals, I must reserve time for me, for should I falter, all who depend on me will be let down. Therefore, I shall rise with sufficient time to allow for hours of meditation and soul centering. After which, I shall adorn myself in a made-in-the-U.S.A. fashionable, waterproof, breathable, sweat suit with state-of-the-art walking gear. To which, I will attach a heart monitor, fire up some inspirational music, grab the walking weights, and tread briskly for miles; assuring my heart rate remains in its ultimate target range the entire time.

Upon returning home, I shall shower in purified, alkaline, ionized microwater, and then prepare the most important meal of the day. My healthy breakfast consists entirely of 100% organic, all natural, unprocessed, non-fat, free-range, locally grown, high-fiber foods. Further ensuring complete balance, I masticate each morsel 32 times, one for each tooth.

This will be my new dawn, my genesis, my beginning. All will be perfect!

Before the rooster crows, I am gently roused by my ascending, progressive, Tibetan chime, Zen alarm. Noticing the early hour, the stars against the dark night sky, and picturing all I will accomplish this perfect day in perfect order — I jerk my certified organic ivory-colored, imported, Egyptian cotton blanket over my head, slam the snooze button, muttering, "Yick, there's always tomorrow," just like I did yesterday.

A thought crosses my somnolent synapses, "Maybe, this all-or-nothing attitude is overwhelming and holding me back? Would I be more productive if I set more realistic goals?"

Pondering the revelation, I realize that if I did, I'd actually have to change. Why would I do that when everything's perfect?

HANGING OUT WITH A BETTER CLASS OF PEOPLE

For the majority of presentations I conduct, I administer an on-line anonymous survey to get a better feel for what's going on inside the organization. Question number one is, "On a typical day, how would you rate your attitude?"

Respondents choose from five answers:

- Extremely upbeat
- Pretty Good
- Average
- Below average
- Extremely poor

I'll 'fess up to the fact that it's not a very scientific question, but neither do you need to work for NASA to answer it. In a nutshell, it's a fancy way of saying, "How ya' doin'?"

Out of the thousands who have responded, approximately 79 percent have said that their average-day attitude is "pretty good" or "extremely upbeat." In effect, that could mean that you — the person reading this — has about an 79 percent chance of saying your attitude (most of the time) falls in one of those two categories. (By the way, only one percent responds "extremely poor.")

Another way to parse that would be, if we were to ask people to use a one-to-ten scale, with the highest number being "ecstatic," and the bottom being "suicidal;" the regular person on an ordinary day would say, "It's about eight."

Question two rates in the same fashion the attitude of those with whom we interact most often: family members, co-workers, and friends. Here the indicator slides to 52 percent. Using the same interpretation as above, that implies that we feel that, although we'd give ourselves an "eight," we'd label others a "five." (Imagine how much it would deteriorate if they didn't have the pleasure of our charming, upbeat positivity to buoy their sagging moods!)

Finally, question three inquires about, "The attitude of those with whom you come in contact on a daily basis?" That scope involves everyone else we bump into, such as clerks, attendants, or phone reps, in effect the river of population flowing across our paths in a typical 24-hour period.

Using the same measuring scale, we sense that only about 31 percent of "those people" possess a "pretty good" or "extremely upbeat" outlook. To spin that yet one more way, we feel that only about one out of three, or one-third, of everyone we meet has a better-than-average attitude.

In summation, each of us feels we're personally doing pretty well, and the folks in the circles in which we travel are holding their own. However, we seem to be pretty judgmental about everyone else, assuming that they really need to get their acts together (which they are, of course, assuming about us).

The hitch in the get along is that attitude is transparent and contagious. We can spot a "negative person" instantly. His supposed attitude is loudly broadcast via body language, facial expressions, even tone of voice. Were turn those perceptions without thought, making countless assumptions, which we communicate. The drawback is, as evidenced here, we might not be responding to what's really going on inside of *them*, as much as to what's occurring within *us*.

While at the gas station, or bank, or simply standing in line at the grocery store, we have a tendency to assume, "I'm doing okay – but these yokels around me, what's *their* problem?" The deal is they're looking at us, and doing the same thing; creating an infinite, expanding loop of negative feedback.

It can't hurt to judge less and assume better; we'll all find ourselves surrounded by a better class of people, who were actually there the whole time.

A PRIMER ON HOW TO CHANGE HABITS

Most of life is done by rote.

For most of us, alarm clocks buzz the same time every morning. The average grocery store stocks over 38,000 items; yet the standard shopper goes to the same store every week, usually on the same day, and chooses from the same few dozen items every outing. We become brand loyal, eating our meals at approximately the same period every day, leave for work at a uniform time, drive a standard route, and return home at a consistent hour every night. Evenings consist of consuming one of a few "favorite" dinners. Entertainment consists of books or magazines from a few select genres and a stable of favorite authors; or maybe a regular line-up of TV shows, which we watch while sitting in "our usual place," and snacking — or not — on the same foods we had yesterday at the same time. At day's end, we retire at the same time, even sleeping with the same person (hopefully), only to repeat these patterns come dawn.

This is not to suggest we are unimaginative, bland, nor boring; rather to illustrate that we are creatures of habit; no if's, and's, or butt's about it.

Reality is these habits make life easier. Picture the above scenario where every single day consisted of an entirely new routine. Exciting? Sure — for a little while. After that, just plain exhausting.

The downside of a life assembled on a foundation of habits are the "side effects;" those unexpected results of our patterns. Make no mistake however; they are every bit as much a part of the habit as are the results we seek. For example, if I'm bored, I eat. If I'm angry, I eat. If I'm sad, I eat. It's a common routine. It allows me to feel better fast. After all, chips or ice cream not only alleviate boredom, but also go a long way toward holding negative feelings at bay — for the short term. The side effect is a weight gain. I get to feel good quickly, for the simple price of obesity long term.

Conversely, some people read a book when bored; when sad, call a friend; and when angry, take a brisk walk. (There is a clinical term for such folks: "Skinny.") Whereby their habits also provide comfort, the side effects are healthier. Should I long for such results, I must also develop similar habits.

The thing is that it's extremely difficult to "drop" habits. Since their sole purpose is to fill voids, simply abolishing them make those holes more painful. This in turn, triggers the very behavior we were trying to banish — which puts our actions at odds with our feelings. In a case like that, emotions almost always win out and the habit — and its side effects — strengthens.

To break this cycle, one must replace the offending behavior with a counterproductive one. So, rather than saying, "I won't eat when stressed," develop a plan, such as, "I'll take a walk when stressed." Providing you don't also grab a candy bar on the way out the door, the anxiety is still diminished — without the pesky side effect. Yes, feels awkward at first (because it's not yet a habit), but given a few repetitions, it eventually forms a new, healthier, habit.

We never really get rid of habits. We put them in cold storage; we can thaw them out whenever we choose. Unfortunately we do that more times than we consciously choose, which is yet one more habit we can change.

THE POWER OF INTENTION

Being a news junkie, I'm glued to the cable networks. Wedged between the peccadilloes of badly behaving starlets and inappropriately tweeted photos, the anchor brings in two political panelists to discuss the upcoming election (Already? Really? Oy!) To feign "balance" he has a GOP strategist and his Democratic counterpart (as if there are only two sides to a story – but don't get me started). I don't remember the first question, and frankly, it doesn't matter; but what I do recall was once the argument commenced, it became animated without delay. Lots of energy and of course, disagreement, exchanged between the duo.

It could have been either one; but in this case it was the GOP guy who started "powering" over anything stated contrary to his position. When the Dem countered, the Repub would shout him down, yelling ever louder. He didn't call names; he wasn't condescending; and – to be honest – he made logical sense (although I disagreed) .But this is not about politics.

After the "discussion" ended, I had a mental image of him talking to his friends off-camera. They were probably all high-fiving, shouting, "Wow! You blew him out of the water," or "He couldn't hold a candle to you." Congratulations would abound; backslapping would ensue.

That's when it dawned on me; his *intention* – as far as I could discern – was NEVER to have a discussion, but rather to prove his point; and that's what showed.

The number one law of change: Intentions direct actions.

When a client asks for advice, my first reply has become: "What's your intention?" Almost nothing matters more in one's actions or communications than understanding that unassuming question. Unfortunately, most of us do not take the time to dig deep enough to analyze that. The result is we find ourselves in a most unhappy place.

Let's take a simple example. You're upset by someone else's comments. Your feelings are hurt. So, you decide that you "need to talk to her." That's fair; and if done well, it's even "healthy." But if the *intention* of what you're trying to achieve isn't clear to her, you'll get in hot water. If the intention is to "give her a piece of your mind," your communication will be much different than if it is to better understand what she meant, or to heal a rift. If you are looking to minimize the chance of conflict and actually accomplishing something, slow down long enough to understand the intention (preferably BEFORE opening your mouth; but it's never too late).

This is because attitude transmits louder than words. A popular study went so far as to say that what we say accounts for less than ten percent of our communication; it's tone and body language (attitude) that matter most. In effect, we might be able to massage what we say, but it's a heck of a lot harder to mask what we feel.

We can apply this same principle to our own actions.

When trying to change a habit, it's imperative to first analyze what is the *intention* of the offending behavior. What does it get us by continuing it – and what is the resultant cost? Once we realize why we we're doing it —our intentions — our next question can be "How do we achieve those goals without the unpleasant side effects?"

Every behavior is born of positive intention; one designed to make our lives easier. Unfortunately, if we don't look beneath and understand those intentions, we can create a mess, even if that wasn't what was intended.

The New Normal

$$\infty$$

I've had a revelation.

Since the "great recession" of 2008 (which appears to still be in process) came trampling through our economic landscape, I have been — like so many others — waiting and hoping for the rebuilding. When will things get back to how they were? Can we soon return to easier times of job security and stable wages? My ship is weary of white caps; I long to navigate calm seas. When can we be there?

While pondering such issues, it fell hard on me, like a load of gold bricks sold on many radio talk shows as a "hedge against hard times." The economy — and our lifestyle — will NEVER return to how it was. The "good old days" (such as they were) are in the rear view mirror and we have no reverse gear. We cannot turn around and they will not come back.

That's an upsetting— some might say "terrifying" — concept. Never again will we be able to conduct our lives and businesses like we did "back then." What we are now experiencing is — and will continue to be — the "New Normal." Until our last days, and those of our grandchildren, "different" will be "ordinary." Future generations will study the heyday of the 1990s and early 2000s much the same as we picture the gay 1890s or the early 1920s; wild, excessive, booming — and only imaginable as images in history books.

I don't mean to be a downer, but it's time we bow to an ever-apparent reality and accept facts for what they are, not what we long for them to be. Denying the obvious delays the inevitable, which furthers great hurt and denigrates our lives. Striving to maintain an illusory status quo by rejecting reality prolongs its effects; and makes worse the pain.

Having said that, I do pride myself on being positive, while understanding that the set up of this column might appear less than optimistic. Yet, it can be. Due to this unhappy situation in which we find ourselves mired, we are becoming more resourceful, better planning our expenses, accepting gratification in that which we took for granted previously, and we are contributing more to our local communities.

These are wonderful changes. Many considered getting "more involved in our communities" or "cutting back on frivolous spending" numerous times before. However, until now, the pressure was not convincing enough to force action. "One of these days…" has arrived. It is today.

Significant change is always born of fear, force, or pain. No one gets up one morning, totally content with life, and says, "Let me see how I can change it." Rather, when circumstances become too uncomfortable, we decide to do something different. The great recession has inflicted much fear and great pain, and has forced upon us harsh change. Although things will never be as they were, we overlook that they can be better. We will have tools and techniques never before considered. We will at some point re-establish equilibrium. Our world will forever be altered; yet it will also be unique with a new set of advantages and benefits; unknown to us today, but surely waiting over the horizon.

The quicker we accept that there is no turning back, the speedier we will face the future — and the faster we will experience these new advantages.

Some might disagree with my analysis; I accept that. However, should I be off track — and society does return to "how it was"— there's is no down side, for if we adjust, we will be healthier and stronger for having worked together and supported each other through these times.

Dog teaching man

I've heard tell that dog owners (or "guardians" as some prefer) look like their dogs. I did not realize with how much haste that transpires.

We have been considering adopting a dog for a few years. As with any important project, we began by identifying what we wanted. One, he must be a rescue dog. Two, she must not be bothered by our two cats (of course how they respond to the dog will be their decision). Three, we wanted a smaller dog that had some personality but was not hyper. Those were the "must haves," the remainder were "would likes." We surfed websites, monitored our newspaper, and checked shelters and animal control with regularity.

Welcome "Jack." He's a five-year old mini-Schnauzer with a persuasive, mostly subdued personality who loves our backyard, follows me like a shadow, is housebroken (yay!), and even understands some commands, allowing me the option to train him even more; something I wanted. While I write, he has already taken to lying in his bed, apparently content to watch me type. (I guess he's hard-pressed for entertainment.)

As for similarity— although I did not think of it when I picked him up; he already resembles me (or I do him). His hair, although dark of base, is basically "silver," slightly disheveled, and he sports a gray goatee in need of a shave. More striking is that he is also into yoga; I've seen him doing "downward facing dog" repeatedly. (Insert rim shot here…)

The one attribute of which I am NOT fond is that, although he slept through night one without incident, he is evidently an early riser, quite contrary to myself. A perk of self-employment with one's home as the office, is the ability to grab a few extra winks each morning, since my commute consists of four stairs. Alas, I fear those days have passed, as Jack is part rooster, prone to rise with the sun (especially ill-fated since this is summer and first light is unfortunately early).

Therefore, today, I awoke far earlier than was my pattern. My wife, snickering wickedly, commented, "Looks like your days of staying up late are over."

Growling (yet another similarity with a dog), I dragged my carcass from my bed to begin this new, unexpected routine. Change had once again scampered into my life, this time in the form of a twenty-pound canine that could not wait to take a walk. "I must teach him the command, 'sleep,'" I wearily lamented as I secured him in his harness.

But that's the way it is, isn't it? We make our plans and move forth into the yet to come. We believe we're in control — but it's illusion. Life steers; we are passengers. Whether changing how we eat, seeking mental health, developing relationships, financial planning, or simply adopting a furry friend, the results of our actions cannot always be predicted nor controlled.

So, once again, I am fine-tuning to the unexpected, a progression without end, and one in which we all engage non-stop. Sometimes, the adjustments are painful; other times, thank God, they are minor. Yet it is unavoidable.

I detest getting up early; it fouls my mood.

But, conversely, I can be buoyed by the outpouring of warmth from this newfound community of "dog people," which has already been as heartwarming and loving as the joy elicited by Jack when I reach for his leash and we head out into the (too early) morning. It's my choice.

Now, which one of us is really training the other?

COMPLAIN, COMPLAIN, COMPLAIN…

My, but we've become a grouchy lot, haven't we? Maybe it's climate change, or the economy; who knows? It could be the alignment of the stars for all I know, but we've got our cranky pants hitched on and we're wearing 'em a little too snug around our sensitive parts.

Okay, maybe YOU are not cranky, but many of us are, and if you won't own it, I will.

I'm at the supermarket loading up on low-calorie, high-fiber, sugar-free, non-fat, no-taste foods that I force down my gullet in order to keep my weight in check. I really want chocolate, french fries, and chips; but that's not happening, so I'm feeling deprived. Adding insult to injury, I don't have time for this errand, but since my refrigerator resembles an arctic cave, I'm cooling my jets in the check out line. The lady in front of me waits until after the clerk has totalled all her groceries before she takes out her checkbook, enough of a trigger to kick my internal curmudgeon into overdrive, "Hey lady!" the voice in my head screeches. "You didn't realize you were going to have to pay for this before hand? Couldn't you have check ready when you got in line… besides you've never heard of debit cards?!!" Since I won't comment out loud (I'm too "polite"), I roll my eyes, exhale with exasperation (making sure she hears it), shift my feet restlessly, cross my arms, and set my attitude to low burn.

Or have you ever had your cell phone drop a call? Jeeze! That irks me! It wasn't even a particularly important call, and to be honest, I didn't want to talk to him anyway, accidentally selecting ACCEPT instead of DECLINE because the layout of the phone is so stupid. Nonetheless, I'm now heavily vested in commiserated about how his 62-inch 3D TV's glasses suck. Really? That's your grievance? There are people who would love simply to witness a sunrise, and you're grouchy because your nifty cool absolutely amazing invention doesn't come with rechargeable batteries? I mean, come on! Yet, I'm empathizing — at least until his call explodes in a burst of static and I detonate a blast of curse words at my phone, cellular carrier, and even the government for allowing such inferior systems to get to market.

Time for a chill pill; on the grand scale of life, most of what rankles us is not even a blip on the radar screen of "real" problems; it's microscopic. Half the time, we don't even remember it long enough for it to survive the ride home, let alone why we got so upset in the first place; yet we're singing "ain't it awful" with the volume on full.

I've got a phone in my pocket that connects me to anyone on the planet, lets me watch family movies, listen to music, and take photographs. It's got more power than the entire computer system on the Apollo space crafts; and I have the gall to launch a hissy fit because I have to push REDIAL? Or I complain about having to drop a few pounds — while half the planet would beg for what I throw away? Spoiled, you're table's waiting.

We don't live in a golly-gosh-gee-willikers fog of happy thoughts and pink ponies; I'm not saying that either. Sometimes, life is tough, sure. But equally true is that most of our "problems" are better than what most of the people on most of the planet face most of the time.

For that I need to be mostly grateful.

COMPETITIVE EATING

If you normally read my columns at the breakfast table, I strongly recommend that you put down your egg white omelet and tofu bacon before continuing. Some referenced cuisine might result in loss of appetite.

Okay, I've warned you; here we go.

My irk-meter is red-lining today. The reason? Something I recently discovered, referred to as the sport (?) of "Competitive Eating. Major League Eating, "MLE," the organization responsible for inflicting upon us these gluttonous, gross, gobbling games is — according to their website — "the world body that oversees all professional eating contests. The organization, which developed competitive eating ... helps sponsors to develop, publicize and execute world-class eating events in all variety of food disciplines."

At the Fourth of July hot dog eating contest, an annual extravaganza, the winner stuffed more than four dozen tube steaks (with buns) down his distended gullet in less time than it takes me to make a pot of coffee. It gets better — or worse, you choose. The buns can be coated in water before consumption, allowing them to become slippery, for ease of entry no doubt. Nothing says "fine dining" quite like meat entrails in a doughy, gooey mass driven into distended bellies at lightning speed.

Don't care for hot dogs? The winner of the hamburger "Square Off" gobbled 93 burgers in eight minutes and a major pizza chain's

"Chow-lenge" led to six one-pound calzones being polished off in six minutes. If you care to inhale a somewhat more refined cuisine, there is a Gyoza competition (2008 record: 231 in ten minutes). How about oyster eating? The record holder here — a woman — chugged 552 in ten minutes; virtually one per second! If the thought of so many slimy, slippery, shellfish slithering past your esophagus doesn't trigger your gag reflex, I've got one more.

Ladies and Gentleman, start your silverware please! Welcome to the Rocky Mountain Oyster championship. In case you are un-aware, Rocky Mountain Oysters, also referred to as "prairie oys-ters," have no relation to the genus Crassostrea. Instead (this is the part I warned you about), it is the term for edible offal, specifically buffalo or bull testicles. Granted, they are usually peeled, coated in flour, pepper and salt, sometimes pounded flat, then deep-fried; but you can prepare it any which way you please — call me small-minded — but I'm crossing my legs while writing.

So why am I so hounded by competitive eating?

I horrified myself by watching some of the videos of these events and it appeared to be a line of "contestants" pounding food into their mouths, with both hands, while restraining the urge to vomit. All the while, the commentator — in awe — jabbered enthusiasti-cally about how the human stomach is not made to hold that much food. "This is amazing!" he said on several occasions, commenting how the participants had to adjust their postures just to allow the food to fit inside them. I understand that it's their bodies. They can abuse them if they wish. I've done my own fair share, so who am I to judge?

What really struck me was the waste. In fairness, much of the money is donated to charity. And I risk coming across to some as crotchety, yet wouldn't it make more sense to give those 48 hot dogs or 200 plus oysters to families who really needed them, while finding other methods to raise funds?

I can (almost) get past the thought of consuming a platter of Mountain Oysters, but I cannot overcome the image of so much wasted food while so many are in need.

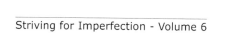

HANDLING THE FOOD ADDICTION

He was celebrating four years of sobriety. When I asked how he knew it was time to initially seek help, he said, "I finally realized I had no control over alcohol. I thought about it all the time. I couldn't wait to drink. I was obsessed with it." As I listened, I thought, "Substitute the 'food' for 'alcohol,' and that's me." It was one of the triggers in getting me to lose my weight.

It was also the instant I realized that overeating is every bit as much of an addiction as drugs or alcohol.

We don't like to think of overeating as an addiction for several reasons. First of all, it's part of the norm to eat too much. That would make us a country of addicts, and true as that might be, we sure don't want to admit it. Moreover, there are no age restrictions, you can do it in public, and it's legal. Eating too much might make you fat, but a cop won't pull you over for a 300 triglyceride level, it won't cause you to black out, nor do unwise things you'll regret with morning's light.

Merriam-Webster's Medical Dictionary defines addiction as, "persistent compulsive use of a substance known by the user to be physically, psychologically, or socially harmful." Let's be clear; when you're hiding goodies in your purse, lying on the bed to tighten your belt, or avoiding social gatherings because you're afraid of the reactions; it's a safe bet you've met the entry qualifications for addicted.

The bigger problem is, unlike the more nefarious addictions, we cannot "just say no." As difficult as it might be, an alcoholic can swear off booze, and a smoker can refuse cigarettes. We, however, must continue to indulge while learning to set arbitrary, always shifting, sometimes ill defined limits about what constitutes "too far."

Sure, a half gallon of ice cream is a pretty clear violation of self control. One could say the same for a quart, maybe. But where do we draw the line? Is a cup all right? What about two? To the alcoholic, an ounce is too much. For us, where does it start?

Let's set the stage: A healthy, thin person consoles herself after a rough day with "chocolate therapy," downing a pint of fudge brownie-chocolate chunk ice cream and a couple of devil's food cookies as a chaser. After sharing with her co-workers the next day, they all laugh knowingly.

"I've been there," says one, "Sometimes, you just need to go with it."

No one thinks she's addicted. She looks great. She's healthy (albeit sporting a humongous sugar buzz). Yet, when I do the same actions for the same reasons, I'm out of control?

See, it's not really about the overeating, but the internal dialog. A healthy personality analyzes the calorie overload and thinks, "Well, that was over the top. I better cut back tomorrow" — and she does, regaining her balance.

The food addict blows it out of proportion, thinking, "Oh my God! I blew it! How could I do this? This is awful! I can't believe what an idiot I am!" Berating her very worth as a human being she finally decides she's a complete failure. With that observation, she gives herself permission to let herself totally go and accelerates over the cliff.

Yeah, we've got issues. Yeah, it stinks. But handling mistakes is part of the process. If guilt and shame were motivational, we'd be skinny as rails. It's not about perfection. Everyone slips up; success will be determined in how we handle it afterwards.

A GOOD TIME THAT DOESN'T INVOLVE EATING

I hadn't seen him in years even though we live in the same town. You know how it is, I'm busy, so is he. Time got away from us. It's not like we had a disagreement, or we didn't want to see each other; it's just that, well, life kicked in…

I answered the phone, "Hey Scott," says he, "I just realized that we haven't gotten together in a long time and we've got so much to catch up on. I thought we could schedule a time."

"Sounds great," I replied, "I can do lunch next Thursday. If that doesn't work, we could get coffee in the afternoon, or, on Wednesday, we could meet early and grab a bagel. Where would you like to go?"

He responded, "You know the park with the duck pond?"

"Yes, the one with all the trails?"

"Yeah, that one. What about Thursday at noon?"

"Sure, that works for me. But I'm not familiar with any restaurants there."

"There aren't any. I've been trying to get in shape, and I know you're always watching your weight, so I thought we could walk and talk. It would be nice to catch up outside."

And so we did. But, can I be honest? It felt really weird; kind of like wearing someone else's clothes. It seems normal enough at first glance, but you just can't get comfortable.

I mean, think about it, what's one of the first questions we ask when we decide to meet up with someone: Lunch or coffee? If you really wanted to crash our economy, ban meetings in restaurants or coffee houses.

I'm sure it goes back to primitive times. It's conceivable (at least to me) that early Australopithecines at day's end gathered around a half-devoured gazelle and discussed their events on the plains. After all, a leisurely grunting session with some close hominoids after a long period gathering, scavenging, and escaping from carnivores would be welcome.

Although the evolutionary train has pulled out, our habits have not. We celebrate with food. We do business over dinner. Relationships begin — and end — at restaurants. Even our last tribute, the wake, is deeply intertwined with eating.

There's nothing wrong with these; don't get me wrong. But one has to admit, that for most of us, it's hard to picture doing anything else with each other. If we're looking to adjust our collective waistlines and get in shape, maybe we need to examine some options. After all, there are book clubs, quilting circles, or even video games.

My son was in town; this usually involves copious amounts of food. Under the television lies our unused video console; the wireless type specializing in sporting events, where one creates icons to compete against each other.

Said he to me, "Bet I can take you in a sword fight."

I might be 30 years his senior but I still have testosterone; I couldn't let that stand.

Our characters faced each other. The battle was joined. After several close rounds, lots of laughter, a great deal of sweat, and exclamations of "You're toast!" or "Take that," age indeed triumphed over youth.

More important, I can already tell it will be one of my favorite memories, far more than yet another trip to yet another restaurant. Plus the added bonus is I got to show him he'd still better not mess with his old man. (Of course, I still can't lift my arms; but I'll deny it if you tell him.)

THE UNLIKELY DINNER PARTY

Some flavors are just not intended to coexist.

Yet my universe happily expanded when someone presented me a french fry dipped in a chocolate shake. At first hesitant, I accepted the offer and discovered yet another tasty food combination dangerous to my diet. This launched me forth on an internet journey in search of other uncommon food combinations or tastes. The result? Yuck; I'll pass. Yet, not wanting to prevent you from making your own decision, please picture with me a dinner party for the "culinarily adventurous" comprised entirely out of actual flavors available to those with strong palates.

While the guests mingle, they nibble from a party bowl brimming with Pickle Jelly Beans, inspired by the Harry Potter series (causing me to wonder why it's so popular). If they choose, they can also snack on other Potter-inspired flavors such as Earthworm, Earwax, Rotten Egg and — I kid you not — Vomit.

Such flavors might turn some away; so as any good host, options are available. That's where Sapporo Caramel comes in, the unlikely marriage of beer and caramel in one effortless sweet. "Candy is dandy but liquor is quicker," said Ogden Nash. Someone obviously took that to heart: Voila! Warp speed.

Once the banquet gets underway, our visitors have a option of two out-of-the-ordinary treats. First up is Baked Pineapple Spaghetti— a creamy, cheesy Punjabi-inspired Indian dish with fruit on top. I can almost see these teamed into one; certainly more than I can get ready for Chocolate Sushi — a Japanese/Korean-influenced dish that pairs eel with chocolate sauce. I love chocolate. I really like Sushi. Yet the union gives me pause; it would be like combining marshmallow crème with salmon. Separated? I'm on board. Together? Not so much.

What's to drink? How 'bout Mashed Potato Soda from Jones Soda Company? I've never met a potato I didn't like, but the thought of a fizzy version of my favorite tuber is a bit hard to swallow (so to speak). Jones also provides a sports-oriented line of sodas to honor the Seattle Seahawks NFL team. Tastes include Perspiration, Dirt, Natural Field Turf, Sports Cream and Sweet Victory.

If you have trepidation about the wasted calories of sugary sodas, alternatives are abundant. In Japan, the distributor of Pepsi markets an ice cucumber flavored cola while a competitor sells Water Salad Soda, billed as — you guessed it — a salad flavored soda pop for the health conscious.

Finally, for dessert, let's wow them with an ice cream bar with such choices as Curdled Bean ice cream, another delightful offering from Japan. Comprised of fermented beans that form a paste that looks like slime from a cheap Hollywood horror flick, and "an odor akin to dirty socks;" who wouldn't shout out, "Give me a double scoop!" Of course, for those naysayers, they can choose other exotic ice cream flavors such as Soy Sauce, Charcoal (sic), Squid Ink or the ever popular Raw Horseflesh with — get ready for it — you guessed it, the same ingredient used in dog food swirled through the ice cream.

Once the guests have left and you prepare to retire for the night, forget the all-popular mint or wintergreen flavors of toothpaste; too dull. Rather put a dollop of Curry Toothpaste on your brush and picture that plaque dissolving while you brush. This flavor, thankfully discontinued, is from a Japanese company named Breath Palette, whose marketing slogan is "Put some flavor in your life." If it doesn't work out you can still get Cola, Pumpkin Pudding, or Monkey Banana flavors.

It's the end of a long night; time to get some rest. Tomorrow's a big day, starting with a cactus-persimmon omelet, which if prepared incorrectly comes with its own toothpicks.

DRIVING CHANGE IN A PRODUCTIVE MANNER

Between the covers of the business book currently on my night stand, the author devotes few pages to discussing cash flow or spreadsheets, while much ink is dedicated to changing one's thoughts about money. It is her premise that our income basically determined more by *how* we think than by the actions we take. Of course, those considerations then produce behaviors, which lead to results. Therefore, if we "dig down" and adjust them, we will do what we do in an altered manner. This provides fresh results improving our business.

In effect, change your thoughts; change your financial life.

The barricade is our ol' buddy, Denial.

Thought patterns, much like a river cutting a path through granite, our etched into our psyche over time, with much repetition. To refashion such embedded patterns takes a great deal of effort — and it's not like we're not busy already, right? Besides, "there's always tomorrow."

The author suggests that such transformation only occurs once "we're hit by a two-by-four." Of course, she's speaking figuratively, not literally. (I hate it when people say "literally" when they mean "figuratively." Sorry, pet peeve…)

Let me expand: Suppose you're in a floundering relationship. You didn't get there overnight; it began subtly, "the small things." For example, you don't talk as much. "It's no big deal," you think, "We're just busy right now." That might be accurate; having said that, "something" still feels off. But, you put it to back burner until you have more evidence — or time.

After awhile, your "couple's time" becomes more sparse. You are roommates more than partners, on parallel tracks with no intersections. Logically, you can explain it away. "We've both got so much on our plates; things will get back to normal soon." No action taken.

Soon, intimacy, in all its forms, has become a memory. There is now real distance, even a bit of resentment. Nobody brings anything up; you're not even sure you want to broach the subject. Also, the chasm is now an additional barrier. Oh sure, you're thinking about "making some changes" when things settle down. For now, it's" stay the course."

Then comes the two-by-four: He wants "out."

"I don't even know who you are anymore," he says, in a difficult, unexpected (?), conversation. "We've grown apart."

It's a pattern experienced by millions of couples. Despite the warnings, and their ever-increasing appearances, we are able to rationalize what's going on, while denying what we felt. Therefore, for most, it takes getting slammed upside the head with a brick (again, "figuratively") before we do what must be done. This is in any facet of our lives, from our relationships to diets to finance.

Newton's first law of motion says that a body in motion will remain in motion unless acted on by an external force. In effect, we will do what we do until, painfully; we can no longer deny the results of our actions. Once at that place, we are so overwhelmed, that it seems an insurmountable problem and we remain stagnant in unhappiness.

First of all, it is not undefeatable if we break it into small steps, and engage in them with regularly and immediacy.

That stated, it's still healthier to avoid that unhappy condition by understanding the urgency of emotions when it comes to moving forward. Look at it this way; our feelings are the gasoline fueling the engine; logic is then the steering wheel. Without the first, we're going nowhere. Without the latter, we're out of control. Developing both is essential to leading a happy, well-adjusted life.

WISDOM OF THE AGES

Please mark this date on your calendar as I have a formal announcement to proclaim. Should lengthy horns from medieval days be nearby — you know the ones with the banners that hung from them — I welcome their use. Milestone events of this stature deserve recognition.

Today is the date when I am officially "old." There, I've said it. I own it. I shall take forth my scepter and move on (albeit slowly).

So what happened from 24 hours ago, when I was but a mere happy-go-lucky youngster of middle-age status; to today, now that the Rubicon has been crossed?

Rest assured, this revelation arises not because of my apparently advancing years, nor because I arrived at a particular birthday. Until recently — yesterday, to be specific — I was convinced we never grew old; we simply became wrinkled children. After all, short of an ache here and a pain there, coupled with a somewhat more "distinguished" look around my temples and eyes, I still think of myself as I did thirty years ago. I suppose most of us do.

Moreover, I'm not complaining about the alterations to my appearance. I mean, I'm not Justin Bieber, surrounded by hoards of swooning teens (nor would I want to be). Unfortunately, I am also not Robert Redford (whom I'd prefer to be); but as far as "men of a certain age" go with regards to the "looks" department, I hold my own. Sure, silver might be the most accurate description for my hair — but I still sport a full headfull. So, I assure you it's not a concern about appearance that pushed me into the amphitheater of the aged.

Yesterday began routine. I awoke, showered, dressed, ate, and hopped on my bicycle to face my day. Appointment one: lead a meeting.

Upon arrival, I noticed one of my shoes had a thick, "athletic-type" lacing; while the other had a more formal, thin lace. "Odd," thought I, "What was I thinking?" When I horrifyingly realized it wasn't that the laces were unlike; it was the shoes! I was wearing two completely different shoes; both black (thank God for that), but one informal, casual; the other for dress occasions.

Mortified, I considered riding like the wind back home, making the swap, and returning. Not a chance; people were already gathering.

I considered going barefoot. Dress slacks, tie, no shoes; how would that work? I could say I stepped in mud! Scratch that, no rain today. Maybe, I could use this as a "teachable moment." Those who noticed would be complemented on observation skills. For those who didn't, I would point out we need to be more observant. "That's it! Put it on them!" The idea faded when I realized the cashier at the grocery store or the teller at the bank in my later errands were not looking for lessons from a older bike-riding guy who can't match his shoes.

I asked myself "WWOPD?" (what would an older person do) and with my new wisdom of being aged I realized: "Put it in perspective. Who cares? Get over yourself. It wasn't the apocalypse. No one was dying."

So I went with it. As it happens, others had done the same thing. It's a function of doing too much, not living too long. Besides, I am getting older; aren't we all? Enjoy the ride as long as you can.

However, truth-be-told, as I pedaled home, I was self-conscious; convinced that a woman in a passing automobile turned to her husband and said, "Honey, look at that old guy on the bike. Do you think he knows he's wearing different shoes?"

WHO DO YOU THINK YOU ARE?

I have a very unassuming, quick-thinking question. Don't ponder the answer; just blurt it out. Ready? (Um, that's not the question.)

Here we go: "*Who are you?*"

At first blush, it's such an innocuous query and our replies come by rote. We provide our name. But, in reality, that's not accurate, because my name is not WHO I am, it's WHAT I am called; it's a label.

Okay, take it down a level: Who is — in my case — Scott Marcus?

Well, I could reply, "a man," "father," or even "American." Those are all true — and actually more descriptive than responding with my name. They deliver more detail, but are still painfully vague. One person's "man" creates images of football players, while another's is an accountant, neither of which fit me. Piling on additional descriptors becomes the next step, "56 year old speaker, writer, father of two sons, married, lives in Eureka."

Certainly this constructs a more vibrant portrayal, but it is still soooooo scratching the surface. For example, should I move from my coastal community to the Arizona desert, would I then be a different person? Better yet, am I still the same person I was a few years ago, or do every 365 days establish a new being?

Circumstances change, but that alone does not mean we are no longer who we were; there is a consistency that remains our core. These modifiers therefore, no matter how many we use, are not answering the core issue. Something lacks.

So, why does this matter?

Words, the vehicle by which we think, create images, which we call "perceptions." Each of us develops reflex like responses to those perceptions. So, should I say "filthy rich man" or "homeless woman," we create immediately an image in our mind about who are each of those people. (I know you did when you read them, as did I.) The hitch is we do not see "individuals;" what we envision are our *perceptions* of that class of society. Should you be strolling through Old Towne and view someone you perceive to be, for example, a "homeless man," you create an entire story in your head, BEFORE even meeting him.

This process is not only in action when we see — and label — others. It is also very much in play in how we view ourselves. The words we tap to describe who we are to ourselves affect the images we see about us, portrayed externally to others via our resultant actions.

If I enquire of myself, "Who am I?" And the reply comes: "A clumsy, stupid, moron who cannot do anything right," I create powerful internal imagery, which in turn, generates an emotional state. Those emotions drive our actions. Logically, therefore, if the language is negative, so too will be its result.

More happily, if my answer is, "A fully-functioning, basically happy, honest, caring, contributing member of society whose doing the best he can to love others, make the world a better place, and take care of himself as well as he can;" those result feelings, and their actions, will be vastly different. (Saying each answer to yourself and notice how you feel.)

When greeted at a party, that answer might not be appropriate. However, we'll experience a far healthier and happier life when we can learn to answer our own internal questions in a more positive fashion.

Besides, who would I be if I steered you wrong?

THE NEWEST DIET IN TOWN

You know how you can be totally oblivious to something? Then you catch wind of it; maybe you hear about it from a friend, or you read an article. Suddenly — BAM! — it seems to pop up everywhere! For me, that's the term "gluten-free."

Last week, I knew virtually nothing about the protein found in wheat, rye, and barley. Yet, literally, in the last few days, it appears to be showing up on all horizons. This could be due in part to the revelation that Chelsea Clinton's 500-pound wedding cake was not only the size of a small trampoline, but equally noteworthy, was that it was also gluten free. The sudden (at least in my world) popularity of gluten-free could also be related to the fact that gluten-free dieting is growing in popularity among Hollywood's upper crust (which, of course, would be made without flour).

There are legitimate reasons for a gluten-free diet, most notably the treatment of Celiac Disease (CD), also known as gluten intolerance. This lifelong digestive disorder affects approximately one of every 133 people. For its sufferers, consuming foods containing gluten damages the small intestine, preventing proper food absorption, resulting in symptoms ranging from diarrhea to weight loss, bloating, or malnutrition. There also might be a connection to osteoporoses, and in some cases, lack of treatment for CD has even been connected to cancer. (Some people believe children with autism are sensitive to gluten, and avoiding the protein can improve certain symptoms, although the idea is controversial.)

Going gluten free to shed pounds however is using a steamroller to flatten wheat-free dough. It'll get the job done, but there are much easier ways to do it.

Thinking of trying it? Get ready to read every single, solitary food label on every product you buy. Some must-avoid ingredients are obvious, such as wheat, wheat gluten, barley, or rye. Yet, others are hidden: malt (made from barley) and hydrolyzed vegetable protein (often contains wheat). Oats are indeed an alternative but for some, may cause abdominal pain, bloating, and diarrhea.

The gluten-free diet is no cakewalk, um, er, oatmeal walk. It's plain difficult and is for the truly dedicated. The forbidden food list consists of the more common breads — including white, wheat, marble, and rye. No more lox and cream cheese on bagels either; or for that matter, muffins, croissants, hamburger buns, or scones. Pizza, and pasta become fond memories, as do most breakfast cereals, cakes, pies, and other treats. One positive note is that those following this restrictive diet will never worry about a beer belly. Yep, most beers are made from barley malt, another on the illicit ingredient list.

There are more and more alternatives to many of those foods, and what is allowed is by no means sparse. Chow down on rice, potatoes, fresh fruits, vegetables, eggs, milk products, chicken (not nuggets), fish, and beef. Summed up, unprocessed meat sans additives are great for a gluten-free diet.

Of course, from a practical view, if we ate fresh, unprocessed foods (gluten-free or not), and emphasized fruits and vegetables, we'd probably be healthier, and most likely at our correct weight anyway. However, it doesn't appear to be unhealthy. It's not easy, and it does tend to be more expensive than simply balancing your diet, so if you try it, you might be a bit stressed – especially at first. The good news is wine and liquors are generally gluten-free so at the end of a long day of label-reading, you can still have a drink.

You just never know

Early morning routine: Jack, my dog, and I are taking our walk. His leash is in my hand, my headphones are clamped over my ears; I am absorbed in the back-and-forth of my favorite pod cast. Jack and I; just doin' our thing.

The neighborhood is residential; no major thorough fares, so I'm quite cognizant of the large diesel truck that rattles up next to us and slows down. Matching my pace, the driver waves at me. I assume he's just being friendly so I return the action, figuring he knows me from my decades of living in a smaller community.

He gestures again, this time I recognize he's motioning me to come over. Pulling Jack's leash in tight, we walk on to the street and approach the open passenger window.

The white truck's interior is clean, uncluttered, and modern, with a flat screen in the center of the dashboard. As for its only passenger, he appears to be in his forties, healthy, short-cropped hair, and brandishing a smile as big as the vehicle and as warm as its motor.

Leaning toward me across the center console, he opens, "You probably don't remember me…"

He's correct.

"…About 25 years ago, I applied for a job working for you. You didn't hire me."

"I'm sorry." A slight rumbling of anxiety bubbles in my belly. Is this some form of latent workplace revenge?

"No need to apologize," he quickly adds, waiving away the thought with his hand. "You were very nice and polite. You told me that you thought I was overqualified and that I would get bored, and you felt my talents would be better used elsewhere. I took your advice."

The truck continues its diesel clattering, I move in closer to hear better.

"I wanted you know that I now run this company; it's worth a few million dollars. I'm really happy how things turned out. You were right."

Pleased (and relieved), I respond, "Oh! I'm glad. Maybe YOU should hire ME."

His laugh is warm, friendly, and relaxed. I suddenly feel like I'm talking to an old friend.

"I see you with your wife walking your dog, and I keep meaning to tell you how grateful I am. But it never seemed the right time — until now."

"Thank you for doing so. I'm really delighted it worked out so well. It's nice to know."

Cars line up and are then forced to drive around us, so, as much as I'm now enjoying this unexpected interlude, I'm self-conscious, and figure I better move on. Before I can, he adds, "Sometimes the Lord pushes you in directions through the people you meet. You are one of those people." He pauses and looks me in the eyes. "Thank you."

With that, we shook hands through the window, said goodbye, and the truck disappeared around the corner.

I remained a statue in the road, and reflected on what just happened. I was humbled, uplifted, honored, and — in some way — I had a more pronounced sense of purpose. I don't know how else to explain it.

We never know, do we, when an action we take will affect someone else in a profound manner? We take care of our families, and ourselves, and in between we try to do our best to treat others with respect and dignity, hoping and praying it all turns out well in the end. Once in awhile, we are lucky enough to find out it did.

What we do matters – in ways we might never even begin to know.

"Have to" versus "Get to"

When you put a few middle-aged cerebral-type guys among the tall trees for a few days, the end product is what I call "intellectual camping;" not much activity but a whole lot of in-depth tête-à-tête. Oh sure, we spent time in the river. Yes, there was some hiking. (Actually, "walking in the woods accompanied by heavy breathing and complaints about sore knees" would be more accurate.) But, most of the time was spent in dialogue swirling about issues pressing to men of our age.

Three decades prior, such subjects would have been rooted in careers, women, and music. Our careers — such as they are — are now established. We are each happily married (and therefore appreciate women in a more specific sense) and although the interest in music hasn't left us, the decibels at which it is played are lower and the beat more subtle. Therefore, most of the talk time wove hither and yon through topics of society, politics, philosophy and — since we are all fathers — children.

One of us has a preteen boy with Downs's syndrome who has still not learned to use the toilet. In some ways, his entire family has to live in thirty-minute segments so the young man can always be around a bathroom. My children, like most, were "potty trained" while toddlers and I found the notion of having to take care of an adolescent in that manner to be overwhelming.

Yet, what impressed me was the mindset of my friend as he talked about the rituals they've developed. I'm sure he would rather not still be teaching a boy of that age how to use a toilet. In spite of that, there was neither resentment nor animosity. Quite the contrary, he mentioned how much he has received from his son — as well as the whole experience. He's more patient and loving because of it. But, what stood out most in my eyes was how he phrased his responsibilities; instead of "I HAVE to help him learn how to use the bathroom;" he said, "I GET to help him learn how to use it."

He explained that he has made a conscious decision to replace the "HAVE TOs" in life with "GET TOs." In that slight adjustment of language comes so much power. It might not always be easy but it is astonishingly impressive.

I think that I — like many — sometimes lament my responsibilities instead of embracing them. From my cranky place, I grumble, "I HAVE to pay the bills," or "I HAVE to go to work." And for anyone trying to lose weight, there's the perennial "I HAVE to stop eating so much." By focusing on what must begrudgingly be accomplished instead of appreciating what we get for the effort, we feel at odds with the universe, rather than embraced by it.

By substituting "GET" for "HAVE," the whole context can swing a one-eighty; and interesting enough, so does one's attitude. "I GET to lose weight" or "I GET to pay my bills" is so much more empowering than the tyrannical "HAVE to." I GET to change my outlook. I GET to be more aware of what I say; consequently, I GET to be happier in the end.

I got to learn that from the father of a young man with "special needs," who apparently, is quite the teacher. Isn't it cool what we GET when we're open to it?

WORKING HARD AT RELAXING

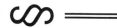

I'm not dead.

At least when I wrote that; I wasn't. Being the intelligent reader of this column, you put two and two together and surmised that in a flash. Hopefully, as you read this, I am still in the not-dead state of being — and shall remain so for decades yet to come.

Having proven therefore that I understand very little about what it's like to die, you will cut me slack about not really knowing — but safely assuming — that no one's last words were ever, "I wish I would have spent more time working and less time enjoying life."

We would agree, wouldn't we?

So, then what's the deal with non-stop, dawn-to-dusk, 24/7, busy-making? We don't ever just "chill." Well, at least I don't; maybe you do, but I'll bet dollars to donuts that you're in the same place. There's so much to get done with so few hours to do it.

Forty-hour workweek; what's that? Wake up. Shower. Shave. Throw some frozen waffles down your gullet while checking the mail and packing lunches. Get the kids to school, pick them up, and beat feet to soccer practice and gymnastics. Straightaway back, homework, meals, brush teeth, and off to bed. To accomplish everything requires groundwork: grocery and clothes shopping, housecleaning, home maintenance, and car servicing. These necessitate steady income — and, oh yes — have you heard the news about the economy? You better not slack off at work or they'll swap you out quicker than a DVD rental on a Saturday night. So, off to the salt mines, bringing our assignments home so we can get them on our kitchen tables in the morning and the bed stands at night. We're work harder while having the privilege of paying more for everything. Come end of day, it's drop like a lead brick off a six-foot wall.

It's no wonder we don't have time for "a life." Or do we?

My sister phones, "What are you up to?" She asks.

I reply, "I'm working hard at relaxing."

Stop the clock. Re-read that response please: "I'm working hard at relaxing." Huh? That statement makes as much sense as "same difference," or "kosher ham;" but I swear it was my reply and I'm betting you relate. Our lives are so cluttered, that if tasks were boxes, we'd be featured on the TV series "Hoarders." No longer are we human beings, we have become "human doings."

Last Saturday, you know what I did? I could have worked on my computer, or mowed the lawn. Goodness know, there were bills aplenty requiring my attention. Nope, didn't do any of those. Instead, I made a conscious decision to do nothing.

It didn't start that way. My dog, Jack, and I went for a walk. Upon returning, he scampered into the backyard, rolled about on his back, feet to the sky; and then did what animals do so well: Absolutely nothing. Zero. He simply "was."

I couldn't remember the last time I did that, so — not having a better plan — I joined him! I didn't put my feet in the air, but I honest-to-God did lie down in the grass and watched cloud animals pass over my head. I felt the sun on my skin. I let my mind go where it went. For a short time, Jack and I simply appreciated that we exist.

Even machines have an off switch. Surely we deserve as much as do they. The world's going to keep on turning, even if you're not the one who's pushing. Take a moment and recharge. You'll get more done later.

WEIGHT LOSS MYTH DEBUNKED

"I'm sorry this article is late; I was going to have it ready yesterday, but the computer crashed and I ran out of toner so I decided to email it, but wouldn't you know; the internet was down. You know how it is…"

From the time we can first speak, we make excuses. Whether it's because we're afraid to appear wrong; don't want to change; really didn't plan on doing what we said; any of the above or all of the above; it's just an annoying fact of the human condition.

There are unimaginative justifications, such as "I was stuck in traffic" or "My alarm didn't go off."

There are I-really-don't-want-to-go-to-work excuses (referred to as "calling in sick"). By the way, should you be in need of an all-around pretext, there's always, "I've got that thing that's going around." (Not that I'm advocating dishonesty mind you…) The cool thing is there is *always* "that thing that's going around." Call in any day, any time of year, make use of that ploy (cough and sneeze for emphasis), and the person on the other end will most assuredly reply, "Oh, yeah, my brother/uncle/husband had that thing. It's awful; it hung on for weeks." No one ever knows what IT is; yet we all know IT, and fear we will get it.

Diet excuses are the most common. As example "I had to go to a restaurant so I didn't know what I could have," implying I therefore ate everything I could. At year's end, "I'll wait until the holidays are over before I start my diet," becomes the conventional understanding.

This of course, ignores the fact that the holidays have been going on for about 2,000 years and show no sign of ending any time soon. Yet, we accept the rationale.

Among career dieters, there is the oxymoronic, "I gained because I'm not eating enough," appearing to make as much sense as "I'm wealthy because I didn't earn anything."

To be fair, this is based on a well-worn dietary concept called "set points." Roughly stated, the theory claims that if we drop too much weight too quickly, or lower our caloric intake below a certain level, our bodies react in primitive fashion, shifting into "starvation mode" as a protection against a perceived famine. This causes our metabolism to slow, allowing us to store energy (fat) for the expected rough times ahead. Therefore weight loss suffers. It does appear to make good sense, and it also provides cover for those few extra chocolate cookies. Beyond that, it's a great scapegoat when we believe that we're really working hard with minimal results. Alas, it has recently been debunked.

It is true that cutting one's caloric intake *drastically* (never a healthy method to lose weight) makes the body more efficient and causes it to lower its metabolism. However the upshot is slower weight loss, not a reversal of it. (Upon achieving a healthy weight, our metabolism returns to its previous state.) While there is no biologic evidence to support the "starvation mode" myth, there do appear to be behavioral explanations as to why weight loss stops from extreme dieting. Over-restriction of calorie intake, known as "high dietary restraint," has been found to be tied to periods of overeating, which of course get in the way of successful weight loss. In effect, we become so ravenous, we pretty much eat anything — and then rationalize the indulgence by the periods of deprivation.

If we focus on long-term health rather than quick-loss diets, not only might we actually drop a few pounds, but a whole lot of excuses too.

IN ONE LIFETIME, WHAT CAN BE ACCOMPLISHED?

If there were neither barriers nor obstacles from birth until death, what could one person truly do in his or her time on Earth?

Over one person's life span, he could build understanding between countries, generating bonds among millions. Should he choose the healing arts, one soul could cure millions on multiple continents, elevating especially the elderly and the young. One man, or one woman, could raise populations from poverty, or tutor multiple generations to read, enlarging possibilities well beyond his days. In one life cycle, great inventions will be created, political movements will be forged, wars might be averted, and peace could take root. One person, one lifetime, with so much possibility...

Yet, what if there was but one decade? In ten short years, what could one person do?

In that period, a parent can raise a child from healthy adolescent to well-adjusted, successful adult; or guide her from a "spark in her daddy's eye" to a happy buoyant, bouncy, smiling, joyful young girl. In 3,600 days, one being can decide what matters, embark on an educational voyage, advance to premier heights, become recognized for accomplishments, and utilize those skills to develop her life — and those of all she touches. She could construct miraculous vaccines, produce rousing movies, pen prodigious literature, or travel the globe and advance deeper understanding of vastly unalike cultures. Should one person choose, even without education, he could opt to support the unfortunate, instruct the uneducated, or comfort the afflicted. In the next ten rotations about our Sun, history could — and most probably will — be affected by one person many times over.

Should you only have one year, what might be altered?

Between now and this date next time, you could reconnect with far-flung family with whom you have lost touch, bringing back a sense of closeness too easily forgotten. In 365 days, you could learn to play an instrument, acquire a language, donate regularly to a cause, or enhance your relationships. In one brief year, you could help mend your neighborhood, volunteer at a school, understand another culture, read great novels, plant a garden, or lose that extra weight and become more fit. One year, a blink of an eye, is loaded with potential. One person, one year, with so much possibility…

In one month, how could things change?

Before you turn the calendar, you could choose what matters most and devote time each day in its pursuit. Should you fancy, you could learn yoga, kick-boxing, water color painting, or cooking. In that time, you could go berry picking, finish painting the house, read several novels, make a movie on your computer, enroll for classes, get caught up on your filing, pay some bills, clean the "junk drawer," donate 30 hours to the homeless, learn CPR, stack wood, plan the best vacation ever, take daily walks; and still have time left over to hold your wife and call your kids (or vice versa). There is so much that can be done in four short weeks.

In one day, what could be changed?

Before tomorrow rises in the east, you could sit in the sun, call a friend, take a walk, write your congress person, start a journal, go to the library, wish well every stranger you see, stop putting off a doctor's appointment, give a few bucks to the guy with the cardboard sign (realizing it could have been you), or leave a happy-face note for your wife.

If you only had "right now," what would you do?

One person, one moment, with so much possibility…

END FAT TALK WEEK

"Say the word and you'll be free."

"Have you heard the word?"

"What's the good word?"

Being a writer and a speaker, I would be the last person in the world to say words don't matter. They do, many times more than we imagine (and often time, more than we think). Words can stab more painfully and deeper than any knife, or they can elevate and lift higher than the clouds. A clever turn of a phrase can be the catalyst for everlasting, uplifting change; or the callously stated, thoughtless verbal venom that spews forth from the lips of an unthinking Neanderthal can generate decades of self-loathing and fear.

Since the medium by which we think happens to be words, it is not a major leap to the realization that our thoughts matter even more than the words we mouth. Born from that unceasing internal dialog between our ears comes motivation to change, desire to act, or justification to quit. It is the birthplace of achievement or the graveyard of failure. Every action taken or avoided began as electrochemical impulses fired across narrow synapses. This in turn formed thoughts, which begat the word, and thus produced our lives. We stand here, each a testament to the words we have told ourselves over time.

Whatever we will accomplish — or will not — will begin or end via the power of the Word. It matters.

So, I was intrigued when I discovered "End Fat Talk Week." I was unaware of such an event, but was thankfully wasting time on social media sites when I stumbled upon it. In light of my interest in weight loss and speaking, I was compelled to delve deeper into this event (to be observed October 18-22, 2010).

Quoting from their fan page (or business page, or Facebook page, or whatever it's called), End Fat Talk Week's mission is, "we believe that by eliminating fat talk, we can start to change the conversation about body image."

As for their description of what is "Fat Talk:" "[It] describes all of the statements … that reinforce the thin ideal and contribute to women's dissatisfaction with their bodies. Examples … include: 'I'm so fat,' 'Do I look fat in this?' 'I need to lose 10 pounds,' and 'She's too fat to be wearing that swimsuit.' Statements that are considered fat talk don't necessarily have to be negative; they can seem positive yet reinforce the need to be thin. e.g., 'You look great! Have you lost weight?'"

Body image is becoming more and more problematic with unrealistic expectations portrayed non-stop in the media. As example, your average, everyday, run-of-the-mill super model is between 15 and 22 years old, about 5'8", and 115 pounds. Women no longer have a monopoly on unrealistic body image either. Your standard male model is between 18 and 25, is a touch over six feet tall, and weighs about 150.

Compare this to the reality that average "real woman" weighs about 140 pounds and is about 5'4". The average guy on the street is about 180 and stands about five-nine. Oh, and by the way, the median age of all Americans is 35.3 years old (the highest in our history).

Truth be told, we are not the people we see on television or in the paper; it's time to accept reality. Some will misconstrue that as an excuse to "let oneself go" and give up. This is not the case. Aspire for happiness and health, not unattainable, arbitrary goals.

Being cautious of our words, and elevating our discourse (internal and external) to a place where we honor who we are, not who we look like, will not solve the problem. However, it is a worthwhile thing to do — all year long.

Stupidity in the Quest of "Skinny"

In the sixties, the main diet methodology was a purple collection of mimeographed pages covered with a lengthy list of foods and their calorie counts. Dieters were instructed to eat only 1,000 calories. Not knowing how to manage our eating (or we would not have been fat), we'd scarf down our daily allotments before lunch and were then faced with two most unhappy options: a) starve the remainder of the day, or; b) quit. Either way, the process was unsuccessful.

Frustrated, many opted for easier fad diets; "The Grapefruit Diet," "Egg Diet," and "Watermelon Diet," to name a few. Same results.

Time marches on but stupidity is eternal; so many continue to engage in diet foolishness. Let's take a tour of some of today's more bizarre diets. (I did not make these up.) As they say, "Do not try these at home."

We'll begin with the *Vision Diet*, based on the logic that if something looks bad, we're disinclined to eat it. So, don a pear of blue-tinted glasses all day and everything you plan to eat will look disgusting.

The flaw? Well, aside from the fact that you could hurt your eyes from wearing tinted spectacles too long, the hole is that — for those of us who overeat — we aren't overly concerned with food's appearance. Let's be honest. When you're gobbling down handfuls of three-day-old leftovers at midnight while standing in front of the refrigerator in your boxers, food presentation isn't them a in criterion by which you're making culinary decisions.

Next is *ear stapling*, whereby surgical staples are placed in the inner cartilage of the ear, supposedly stimulating pressure points that control appetite. (One might assume the constant stress of having sharp objects in your ear would actually cause you to eat.) In actuality, the body shortly gets used to it, so one reverts to old habits — or amplifies the process by adding more, developing an abnormal attraction to office products.

While on the subject of body altering, make some noise for the Tongue Patch, whereby a one-inch square of mesh is sewn onto your tongue. Unlike medical patches, it contains no medicine. Instead, it merely makes it difficult—even painful—to eat solid food, so the dieter literally starves herself. But wait! There's more! For $1,500 or more, you get the further benefits of possible choking and nerve damage. Of course, once the patch is removed, old habits return, albeit with a strong craving to chew on your pants.

Other examples of dietary dumbness include the *Cigarette Diet*; you smoke instead of eat. Total weight loss is determined by how much your lungs weigh upon removal. The *Cotton Ball Diet* involves swallowing cotton balls to fill up before eating. One could accomplish the same objective by consuming paper — while having the added benefit of helping to recycle trash. Feed your sweet tooth with The *Twinkie Diet*. Twinkies, day and night, night and day. Since there is insignificant nutritional value in these not-found-in-nature foodstuffs, you might as well engage in an all-chocolate or all-vodka diet for the same results.

Finally, winning the "most disgusting award" is *The Tapeworm Diet*, illegal in the U.S., but still offered elsewhere. One ingests beef tapeworm cysts, which eventually interfere with digestion and absorption of nutrients, generating significant weight loss. Once goal weight is reached, an antibiotic is given, which kills the tapeworm so it can be expelled. Aside from the "yick factor," other side effects can include cysts in the liver, eyes, brain, and spinal cord with potentially lethal consequences.

However, just thinking about that is enough to squelch one's appetite causing a drop of a few pounds — so maybe it does work after all.

PILOT OR PASSENGER?

Three decades ago, I was music director at a highly rated classic rock radio station in SoCal, when I got an unsolicited call inviting me to become program director of a couple radio stations on the north coast of California. I was packed and out the door before the phone was returned to its cradle.

Originally, I planned to stay "a few years" and then move to San Francisco for large dollar contracts and throngs of adoring fans. As it turns out, such fame and fortunate apparently rank lower than redwoods, ocean, and community. Henceforth Eureka is still my home. I love it. I have no interest in leaving.

At least I didn't — until recently.

Being a speaker, it's easier for me to go to an audience than it is to transport them all to me. Therefore, I rely on airports. My livelihood — as well as my contribution to our local economy — depends on them.

Our modest airport has never been highly efficient. The folks who work there are indeed professional, quite nice, and extremely helpful; a few even know me by name. I like that.

It's also an attractive place, so the environs are appealing. Yet there is this ongoing "fog issue," the result being that one can never be sure if and when he will depart or arrive. To compensate, I fly earlier than necessary and pray a lot. Far from the optimum solution; yet it usually works.

Recently however, due to a mandatory upgrade, approximately 75 percent of flights are being delayed or cancelled. I understand these adjustments are required. Yet, if more flights are off-schedule than on, it appears — just say in' — that something was amiss in the planning. I admit ignorance to having all the details; I understand I am not the airport's only passenger; I realize they're trying to make the best of a bad situation; but this is my busy time of year and it's costing me a small fortune, as well as damaging my reputation for reliability; something I am not sure I can recover.

What this triggers in me is that before I fly, I have become an obsessive red-lining, internet-monitoring, weather-tracking, cloud-watching, overly-nervous compulsive; monitoring every flight-tracking and weather website this side of the stratosphere. I am forever on-lookout for any indication about what will happen so I can inform my client and try and make necessary adjustments.

I worry myself into frenzy. If anxiety were a force of nature, I personally could transform our weather. But, alas it's not. It does what it does, oblivious to my needs. The airline staff resourcefully responds as it can (my heart goes out to what they must be going through). The flights go or they don't. It is all so blastedly frustratingly out of my hands!

In calmer moments, it occurs to me that the real problem is not with clouds, federal mandates, nor airport management; it's my response. Attempting to control that over which I have none is not only wearisome, but an excellent recipe to muck up a perfectly good life.

Sometimes, we get confused, believing we can direct the outcome of events beyond our grasp. Stressing and straining, believing if we can just worry enough, we'll get it done; certainly a fool's errand. We only have power over our own actions and consequent responses. It's infuriating. It's exasperating. It is also reality.

Sometimes we're the pilot, sometimes we're the passenger. Double check your boarding pass before strapping yourself in or you might encounter excessive turbulence.

WOULD YOU SAY THAT TO YOUR CHILD?

The family and guests have retired to the living room after dinner. Heather, just shy of her first year, utilizing the coffee table for support, pulls herself to her feet. This is not the first time; it's becoming a habitual (but always exciting) occurrence. Dad jokes that she's making the transition from "horizontal infant noise unit" to "vertical toddler noise unit."

Focused on taking her first steps, Heather lets loose the table, and like a diaper clad, drunken, miniature sailor, wobbles in place for a moment, attaining her balance; her hands out in front of her pudgy small body for stability.

Realizing this could be "the moment," Mom grabs the flip-camera and starts recording. "Come on Honey!" she says. "You can do it!"

The room becomes silent in anticipation. Whatever conversational stream that had been is no more. All are focused on the one-year-old star of the moment. "Come on Heather sweetie. You're a big girl. Walk to Daddy," says the proud papa. He extends his hands, offering a goal.

Heather, cautiously, and without much steadiness, moves one chubby leg, waits a moment to regain her equilibrium, then shifts the other pudgy foot. She looks up at her parents for acknowledgement, a drooly smile exploding from her chubby cheeks.

"That's my girl! You're doing it. Come on!"

She takes another stride, then one more. Four steps; she's cleared the coffee table. Guests are cooing and laughing. Mom has the camera focused. Excitement is palpable.

As Heather reaches for one more step, she takes a header on to the soft carpet, rolls over on to her back and looks at the adults in attendance. The room erupts in applause. Mommy and Daddy spring from the couch; Daddy lifting the baby girl above his head, and commences twirling her high in the air, as the room chants; "Heather is a big girl! Heather is a big girl." Laughter and clapping rebound off the walls.

Imagine a perverse scenario in a backwards world. What would it be like, if at the end of a young toddler's first few steps, those closest to her opted to insult her for falling so quickly rather than encourage her for the distance she travelled? "You call that 'walking'?" they would say. "If that's all you do, you'll never get anywhere."

Of course, such a horrible situation would never occur. Aside from the moral implications of treating an infant with such disdain, the reality is that — should it happen — the young toddler would never again attempt anything new. She would remain prone on the soft carpet for years, never advancing, stagnant, moribund.

As adults, (despite how we might feel at times) we never really get "old;" rather we become wrinkled children. No matter how many years we have logged, that internal small being without end requires encouragement and support. So, it seems counterproductive — even psychically damaging — that what we would never say to a child we are often times quick to unleash upon ourselves. It's a heartbreaking reality that if we spoke out loud to children half of what we verbalize internally to ourselves, virtually every "mature" adult could be hauled into jail for emotional child abuse.

If personal insults and invective were beneficial, we would each be happier and more successful than we are. They are not. That method doesn't work; never did, never will.

For one week, make a commitment: If you wouldn't say it to Heather, don't say it to yourself. Consider it a first step.

WE ARE ALL CHILEANS TODAY

I am exhausted.

I don't mean eyelids-are-drooping-and-I-have-to-find-a-place-to-put-down-my-body fatigued. A cold shower will be of no value. Neither extra shut-eye nor energy drinks will send this tiredness packing. For this lassitude is a psychic, emotional, soul-draining condition felt deep within one's marrow. Its frosty grip suffocates the heart and — in darker lonely times — feels like a virus has spread through the spirit.

Why would such an optimistic being as myself be laboring under such a burden? I'm not sure; yet I have theories. It's not age; there are a few things I would prefer reversed, but it's no big deal, "comes with the territory," as they say. My marriage is great, thank you. I'm paying my bills, and, especially in light of today's economy, I'm incredibly grateful for that. So, if forced to put money down, I'd wager what's affecting me most is the state of discourse in our great land — particularly in politics.

I've never seen our "leaders" (quotation marks necessary) act with such a prevalence of boorish, childish, self-absorbed behaviors. Granted, politics is rarely a selfless occupation populated with courageous, principled, altruistic individuals willing to sacrifice career for Greater Good. Yet political discourse now, once considered noble and eloquent, has degraded to what one would overhear between bullies in a kindergarten sandbox.

"You're a stupid head!"

"You're a dumbo face!"

"Nuh-uh!"

"Fraid-so!"

"Stupid head!"

"Dumbo face!"

The words are not accurate but the attitude is spot on. Nothing is accomplished; nothing changes. Worse yet, without support, even the status quo cannot hold, it deteriorates. Wars continue. Economies falter. Our planet hurts. People suffer.

Yep, I'm pretty sure that's why I feel so cheerless; I know I'm not alone. Worse, infected by listlessness, everything merits complaints. Life sucks. Work stinks. Even the weather is lousy. It's too windy. It's too hot. It's too foggy. Blah, blah, blah…

As I write this, the miners trapped 70 days in a Chilean mine are being hoisted, one by one, through a narrow tube, from half mile underground, to the loving embrace of friends, family, and an enrapt world. More details will emerge; but this we know: To survive, they supported, encouraged and counseled each other. In a place literally as close to Hell as any humans have ever existed, their better Angels held forth.

As Florencio Avalos, the first to emerge, exited the wire cage that brought him topside, the entire world was Chilean. We felt the embrace of his wife and the relief of his child. We cried tears of joy as he breathed in fresh air for the first time in over two months. We shared the bear hug with Chilean president, Sebastián Piñera; and our chests swelled with pride while the crowd chanted "Chi-Chi-Chi! Le-Le-Le!" With each man's emergence, from 622 meters below the Atacama Desert, we willingly experience it again and again and again.

It just does not get old.

From tragedy has risen hope, like the Phoenix capsule in which the miners rise.

We need to be reminded — I know I do — to be more grateful for what we have. Personally, I might not like the fog, but at least I can hold my wife's hand and walk freely into it whenever I choose.

POTATO WARS

Let us dispel the belief that we have a "do-nothing congress."

Our Senate recently stood shoulder-to-shoulder in solidarity with the lowly white spud, rebuffing an effort by anti-potato Obama administration to limit its consumption by schoolchildren. Before you get the inaccurate image of the president and his cabinet slapping french fries from the hands of kindergarteners, you need to know some details.

The administration had proposed limiting the amount of potatoes and other starchy vegetables that can be served in school lunches to one cup per student per week. Beyond that, they wanted to ban them from school breakfasts entirely.

Imagining the horror of a world where breakfasts are without the crunchy, fatty texture of hash browns; and quicker than a fast food chain can deep fry a basket of sliced spuds, the Senate blocked the proposal by adopting an amendment to the 2012 spending bill for the Agriculture Department. The amendment, approved by unanimous consent I might add, prohibited the USDA from establishing "any maximum limits on the serving of vegetables in school meal programs." Paraphrasing the quotation usually attributed to Voltaire, "I disagree with your choice of Russets but I shall defend to the death your right to eat them."

In this age of hyper-partisan non-stop bickering and political tantrum throwing, it's comforting to know that members of our legislature could reach across the aisle for the common good. (It would be nice if it benefited our economy but one must take the victories he gets. Sigh…) Senators Susan Collins, Republican of Maine, and Mark Udall, Democrat of Colorado, set aside partisan differences and defended the starchy spud— coincidentally grown in great quantities in their states — saying that the proposal had no basis in nutrition science. (Not that has always made a difference in how laws have been crafted previously.)

Said Ms. Collins, "The proposed rule would prevent schools from serving an ear of fresh corn one day and a baked potato another day of the same week, an utterly absurd result."

Why was the potato singled out, you might ask? Well, that's because, unlike celery or green beans, potatoes are defined by the Agriculture Department, as "starchy vegetables." In addition to white potatoes, this category includes the aforementioned corn, as well as green peas and lima beans. (I thought edamame fell within this classification but it turns out it's a legume. Besides, there doesn't seem to be a lot of excitement for a dish of green soybeans boiled or steamed in their pods.) The department's intent in limiting consumption of starchy vegetables was to "encourage students to try new vegetables…" Personally, I believe the bill targeted the potato because I cannot imagine elementary school children queuing up for an extra helping of lima beans. However, I could be wrong; after all, I enjoy edamame.

Ms. Collins, who started as a small fry amid the potato fields of Maine, (insert rim shot here…) pointed out: "Potatoes have more potassium than bananas. They are cholesterol-free and low in fat and sodium and can be served in countless healthy ways."

Mr. Udall said, "Anything can be fried or drowned in any number of fats…" The problem, he rightly pointed out, is not with the potato, but with how it is sometimes prepared. This is true, no doubt.

And I am in firm agreement with the goal of improving the nutritional content of our youth. Also, in the interest of full disclosure, I have been known to accept payment in the form of french fries. Having said that, it's unlikely you'll find the next junk food crazes to be either broccoli chips, or mashed celery slathered in sour cream and butter.

HUMAN GUINEA PIGS

Summer is over; the kids are back in school; vacations have become memories; and more and more folks turn their attention to the task of "dropping those few extra pounds" before the holidays. It is such a widespread phenomenon that the weight loss industry refers to it as, "the winter diet season." Especially during these months, many well-intentioned (but misguided) individuals opt for what they think are "safe and natural" methods that will accelerate weight loss with minimal habit change.

Recently, Abbott Laboratories, manufacturer of Meridia, opted to pull the diet drug from the market after failing to win the approval of a safety advisory panel affiliated with the US Food and Drug Administration (FDA). The latter requested that Abbott withdraw the drug; they complied. At the same time, the FDA warned consumers against a dietary supplement — *Slimming Beauty Bitter Orange Slimming Capsules* — due to its active ingredient, Sibutramine, (found in Meridia).

For perspective, the FDA approved Sibutramine in 1997 for obesity management, including weight loss and maintenance of weight loss (which — I point out — they said should be combined with diet and exercise). Twelve years later, a major study found that patients with a history of cardiovascular disease who took such medications had an elevated risk of heart attacks and stroke, as well as uneven heartbeat and shortness of breath.

What's particularly troubling is that a recent report shows that many supplements, which bill themselves as "natural," are actually laden with laboratory drugs — including some illegal ones.

Researchers in Hong Kong analyzed 81 weight-loss products taken by patients who came in to the hospital for treatment for poisoning (one of which had died). They discovered two or more pharmaceutical agents in 61 of the supplements, and two supplements contained six drugs. The authors caution their findings should not be interpreted as a full analysis of the weight-loss supplement market; yet, it bears noting that in the good ole U.S. of A., approximately $34 billion is spent annually on alternative medicine, including supplements. This equates to about $110 per man, woman, and child per year. Many of these products, sometimes called "botanical supplements" or "herbal remedies," are not well studied according to research published in *Chemical & Engineering News*. In some cases, they note, the ingredients could even be dangerous.

Within the last two years, the FDA has alerted consumers about 72 weight-loss supplements containing such undeclared drugs. In addition to the above-referenced Sibutramine, they found Fluoxetine, an antidepressant best known as Prozac. More disturbingly, a number of them contained banned drugs; including the laxative phenolphthalein, which was outlawed because of an association with cancer. More notoriously, the appetite suppressant Fenfluramine was found in several supplements. As a refresher, Fenfluramine was the "fen" in the Fenphen diet pill, which was pulled from the U.S. in 1997 for its association with heart attacks.

Herbs, vitamins, or natural supplements can be excellent additions to increase one's health. However, it's urgent to remember that "health" is always the top objective, and the most "natural" way to enhance that is to move a little more and eat a little less. It might not be quick, but there are very few side effects.

Radical forgiveness for the holidays

The common, accepted portrayal of a happy, joking, and support-ive family joyously celebrating around a food-laden Thanksgiving table is definitely not a universal reality.

Some families despise the ritual (and aren't too keen on one an-other either); yet they meet year-after-after out a sense of guilt or tradition, jabbing each other with passive-aggressive verbal stabs. Even within families that are indeed content overall, certain mem-bers of the clan might resent, or even dislike, one another. They hold grudges over past transgressions or historic bitterness stalks silently beneath a transparent veneer of tranquillity.

I point out these realities not with intent of injecting an unpleas-ant aftertaste to Thanksgiving dinner, nor as some sort of post-apocalyptic view of the holidays. And to be honest, I also do not know percentages of "unhappy" versus "happy" families; maybe it's minuscule; possibly it's everyone but you and I. Yet it is true. More-over, to focus on "how many" bypasses the greater issue: we cannot release these strains until we acknowledge they exist. Once there, we discharge them with a type of thanks.

"Thanks," you might ask with understandable confusion; "Why would one give thanks for an irritating collection of boorish rela-tions with whom I'm forced to endure boring football games and overcooked turkey?"

In the traditional sense of "giving thanks," you wouldn't. However, when one expands the concept of thankfulness, we realize that gratitude and forgiveness are actually the same act. All that differs is the direction in which they are pointed.

Similarities abound. Each brings with it a sense of inner peace and happiness. The action in each is directed toward another person; yet its true purpose is to help us, not the recipient. Each releases an responsibility: whereby thanks releases me from obligation to you. Forgiveness un-tethers you from a perceived debt I feel you have to me. The results are identical; what differs is the grounds. We give thanks when we believe something is "positive," while forgiving what we consider "negative.

Of course, it's normal to feel someone is unworthy of forgiveness. In effect, I cannot forgive you because the pain you inflicted was so extreme, or because I was so violated, that I lost control over part of my life; in essence you took away a part of ME. How do I forgive such heinous acts while remaining true to my core beliefs?

The dilemma lies in equating forgiveness with approving the behavior.

Forgiveness is actually about my feelings, not your actions. If I change the perspective from "what you did" to "how I feel about what you did," I reclaim control over my emotions and can begin to regain that which was taken. The only alternative is to continue to be a victim, experiencing the anguish on a regular basis — the torment not only extreme, but also constant and repeated.

Unfortunately many view forgiveness as a mark of weakness. The reality is it requires enormous strength to direct one's emotions. Said Ghandi, "The weak can never forgive. Forgiveness is the attribute of the strong." Forgiving what your sister did long ago, or how your parents mistreated you is not easy. However holding longstanding grudges does zero to help heal the pain, and — can we be honest? — it's really not hurting them in the slightest.

It might be time to let go, even a little. And this holiday seems as good of a time as any to start the process.

DOES IT PASS THE SMELL TEST?

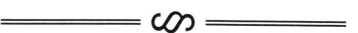

Smell is our most dramatic sense.

As example, it might have been years since losing touch with a friend who always wore one particular brand of perfume. One day, while wandering through the mall, someone passes you adorned in that exact long-forgotten fragrance. As it gently wafts past, you are without delay jolted back to a vibrant, dynamic, long-forgotten recollection. Only the sense of small transports us so fully. Photos bring back images. Recordings make us nostalgic, smell stands alone in its ability to transform.

Smell is so potent and primal a force that it can induce healing, as evidenced by the increasing popularity of scented candles, essential oils, and aromatherapy. Smell can change thoughts or moods; even triggering us to take actions to which we might normally be resistant. Want to get your kid off the couch? No problem. According to researchers, the aroma of strawberries generates an urge to exercise.

While on the topic of a increased activity, suppose your husband or male partner has become lackluster in the bedroom. Re-kindle that waning passion by combining the scents of pumpkin pie and lavender, at least according to researchers. Conversely, they claim that women become more amorous when exposed to the scents of — I kid you not — cucumbers and the candy "Good and Plenty." Husbands, I'll meet you at the produce section; then we'll hit the candy store!

Not wanting to be left behind, diet researchers have discovered that we actually tend to eat more (sic) when food has been altered to have a bad smell instead of a pleasant smell. To me, this seems counter-intuitive, but the results stand. Scientists provided test subjects meals that were sprinkled with "tastants." What they discovered was that when the aroma was enhanced with a combination of green apples and peppermint, people ate less than when the smell reminded diners of dirty socks. (I swear I am not making this up.)

Enter a new diet product claiming to take advantage of our subconscious triggers. The manufacturer claims that to lose weight, all one must do is sprinkle their powdery product on every morsel of food consumed. In the name of easy weight loss, I guess some will consume just about anything as its formula includes silica (found in sand) and Carmine, the latter a derivative of carminic acid, found in insects, who apparently do not part with it willingly. Therefore it is obtained by boiling down dry insect carcasses.

Dead insects notwithstanding, several participants engaged in a six-month study, where they lost an average of about 30 pounds each. I'll admit that's a healthy, realistic weight loss; but I would be remiss to not point out that any healthy eating program would generate similar results. More importantly, in the latter case, the loss would more likely be sustained long-term because the dieter actually changed her lifestyle.

So how does it work? What allegedly occurs is that this product works with your taste and smell senses to trigger the satiety center of the brain, naturally inducing the feeling of fullness. Here's where I have my biggest difficulty. Even if it works and it does provide a sense of fullness, most overweight folks usually do not usually stop eating when they feel satisfied. If we did, we wouldn't be overweight. The reality is we tend to eat more for external reasons, such as emotions or celebrations, than for hunger. So anything that doesn't address that core issue simply does not pass the smell test.

Re-discovering hope

Oops! I made the misstep of watching the news, not wise if you wish to maintain an upbeat attitude. Rather, it's an excellent way to become discouraged.

Politicians, with soft spines and moral compasses no longer pointing north, have become wholly owned subsidiaries of Special Interests Inc. and Mega-Business Unlimited. "Establishing justice, insuring domestic tranquility, providing for the common defense, promoting the general welfare, and securing the blessings of liberty to ourselves and our posterity," has been crushed under the weight of partisan bickering and a landscape awash in uncountable dollars.

There is plenty of blame to share; as they say, "we get the government we deserve." But since money has long tentacles, we seem — in my humble opinion — to be getting the government the upper crust deserves.

I am not a "class warrior." I do not dislike nor inherently distrust the wealthy; truth be told, I would like to be so labelled. I also do not believe that money is the "root of all evil," rather it simply allows you be more of who you already were. As illustration, if you're a charitable, involved, dedicated person with an empty wallet and fate or hard work decrees you great prosperity, you become a charitable, involved, dedicated person with a lot of money; able to do much more. Unfortunately, if you were a jerk with but a few dollars who happens to receive a fortune; you become a jerk with a lot of coin, increasing your jerkness. That said, I cannot deny that — lately — it appears many well-off folks have an "I-got-mine,-the-heck-with-you" way of thinking.

It is distressing to think that the concept of helping "the least of us" has become quaint and passé.

An addict, unable to give up my painful addiction, I collapse on my couch to watch the Sunday morning news shows. Ironically from the same spring as my depression bubbles forth hope.

Warren Buffett, Bill and Melinda Gates, and Ted Turner; three members of the aforementioned privileged order were discussing their views on charity and — in a broader sense — the general order of society. I do not have a great deal in common with these denizens of the uber-wealthy community. They can spend more at a restaurant than I will spend on a year's groceries. I seek out for-sale items in stores they buy and sell. We're not on the same strata.

But short of the number of zeros in our paychecks, turns out we actually have a lot in common. Ms. Gates summed it up, "With great wealth comes great responsibility." All are working diligently to give away vast amounts of their fortunes before they die; Mr. Buffett has pledged to donate more than 90 percent. With projects ranging from U.S. schools to Global Nuclear Disarmament to Energy Conservation, this crew of ultra-fortunate share a belief that we are all interconnected and they are asking others of the same class to join them, sharing a common belief that it is wrong to not give it back to those on whom their success was built.

I understand they are not saints (none of us are). I know they don't have to choose whether or not they can afford to go to a doctor. None will ever wake up at 3AM wondering how to pay their mortgages. Yet, that does not detract from an extremely powerful benevolent gesture.

Maybe, just maybe, we're better than I thought we were. I can hope.

FAMILY HISTORY AT THE HOLIDAYS

At four years old, in 1930, with a mop of brown curly hair, bright hazel eyes, and light skin, Ruth Pinsker waited with her family on the side of a slickened Detroit avenue for a cable car they would never ride. Her family was comprised of Zlate and Shmuel "Sam" Pinsker; two immigrants who had recently migrated to the U.S. from Russia; as well as her younger sisters, Mildred; two years old, and the newborn Eleanor; still swaddled in her mother's arms.

An attorney, driving while heavily under the influence, careened out of control down the boulevard toward Zlate and the kids. Although Sam would have been spared, he instead shoved them out of harm's way, taking the full broadside in exchange and killed upon impact. Zlate was dragged under the auto's wheels, breaking several bones. The children — short of emotional trauma — remained untouched.

Zlate did not speak English, and since the only kin she had in this country was her brother, officials felt it would be "better for all" if the children were removed from her custody while she healed. It took an act of congress to allow her entry into the United States. It would take more than that to get them to take away her children. With the help of the community and friends, my grandmother raised her children from a hospital bed until she was able to leave; becoming a pioneer, one of the earlier women in Michigan to pilot her own business, a junkyard, which survived for decades.

Every family has its history, passed from mother to son, father to daughter, weaving its way through generations and across time.

Obviously, I am unclear how much of what I know actually occurred as I relate it. Families tend to make their backgrounds more heroic and less bland.

What I do know is that Ruth Marcus would have turned 85 this week. Her memory, unfortunately fading, is still a guiding light.

As a young woman, Ruth earned her keep as a radio actress and copywriter. In her sixties, she retired as an executive assistant for the California State University system. She was married once, for 25 years; it ended poorly (I won't go into details). Aside from my sister, my aunts, and myself, her greatest joys were playing the piano (never took training), acting, travelling, and reading. She never went anywhere without a dog-eared paperback in her oversized purse.

What I remember most was her laugh, a rowdy unrestrained explosion of elation. Ironically, the recollection is so strongly charged because she became so angry at me once when I asked her to "tone it down." Our family and the Barabashes were attending a concert at the Hollywood Bowl, Mom and Mrs. B hooting hysterically in the last row of the shuttle bus. Being a teenager, embarrassed by virtually anything my parents did, I rudely request they be quiet because everyone on the bus was looking at them. Bad move on my part…

My mother froze mid-guffaw, her expression transformed from happiness to humorlessness as she faced me down. "Don't ever tell me not to laugh. There are plenty of times in life when we will cry. You never know when we'll get the chance to laugh. Any time you do, take it — and apologize to no one for it."

Families come in all stripes. However, my wish for you during this season, no matter the structure of your "family," is that you share wondrous stories, be of good health, hug much, and laugh often. In the end, that's all that really matters.

GETTING STARTED FOR THE NEW YEAR

There was a cosmic event this week. For the first time in 400 years, one could view a full lunar eclipse on the Winter Solstice. If you were crazy enough (like me), you even went outside in the cold and stared up at a reddish, glowing moon. (What was really a cosmic event was that it was clear enough on the normally foggy Northcoast to actually view it!)

At precisely 12:01AM January 2, another cosmic event shall occur, although it happens annually. Step outside at that moment and you will hear a giant clunking sound rumbling across this wide land as the consciousness of the population shifts from "how much can I indulge?" to "how can I undo what I've done to myself for the last two months?"

To capture this public consciousness, you will be inundated with experts telling you how to stick to resolutions and providing all sorts of tools to assist you in that noble quest. Advertisements for in-home gym equipment will converge on you. Infomercials will scream (falsely): "LOSE WEIGHT WITHOUT CHANGING YOUR HABITS." The back page of periodicals will sport a full-page banners proclaiming: "SECRETS THE WEIGHT LOSS INDUSTRY DOESN'T WANT YOU TO KNOW."

Simply put, these are gimmicks. Remember the adage, "If it seems too good to be true, it probably is."

Reality is that we are where we are because of what we have done so far. Period. If we wish to be somewhere else, we must do something else. No matter how loud the scam artists scream from the rafters, nothing changes if nothing changes.

If one were to look at the construction of our lives in the same way a contractor might plan to build a barricade, things make sense. Each brick is carefully chosen, sized, and cemented in its space. Over time, an entire, structurally sound wall is formed and the structure evolves into a fine fortress, secure in it's ability to prevent intruders. However, it can also hold us prisoner.

Although our bricks are made neither of quartz nor clay, we are architects; our building blocks are the actions and thoughts we have used and reused over the decades. As illustration, the block entitled "celebrate" is often located next to the one labelled "eat." The unit holding down "take a walk" is entitled "stay comfortable."

Resolutions fail because we try and remove too many of bricks at once. "This is the year I'm going to lose 20 pounds, stop smoking, exercise daily, stress less, and spend more time with my family," we proclaim. It's not that these are unworthy or un-achievable goals; it's that they are so interwoven into the wall of our life that we have to demolish the whole entity simply to move forward. To drop some weight, I must re-learn how to celebrate, shop, and handle my emotions. If ceasing smoking is the objective, I must find a substitute when the habit calls, develop support, and learn rearrange my life so a new option is always at the ready. Every change requires a series of others to support it, a cascading effect. Stated else wise, I cannot demolish my wall, I must substitute each brick with a fresh one or my entire existence feels like it has literally fallen apart and I rush quickly to rebuild it.

To get past this Catch 22, think smaller. Resolve to pick the ONE thing that matters most and agree to repeat this action every day NO MATTER WHAT. Once you have cemented that in place, add on to it.

Success is built in small steps; failure collapses all at once.

BICYCLIST VS. CAR

Yesterday was horrible.

I was going to ride my bike to my appointments. The bright sunny clear morning sky cooperated as I headed north on E Street. Upon reaching the intersection of Highway 101, I waited for a green light.

Once it changed, a car heading in the opposite direction proceeded into the intersection, as did I. Yet, instead of going straight, the driver turned on to the highway and directly at me. Unfortunately, the laws of physics say only one object can occupy a space at a time; so when a 2,600-pound car and a 180-pound bicyclist collide at the same point in time, one of them will be moved. Of course, that was me — and in a rather forceful manner.

Upon the horrifying realization that there was no way to avoid being hit, time slowed down. As I saw the automobile come into contact with me, I thought, "My life is about to change." The only unknown was "How much?" As the front bumper impacted my leg, I sent up a quick prayer, "please let this be minor, and if not — please let it be quick."

My bike fell under the car as I rolled on to its hood, smashing into the windshield. I vaguely recall the vehicle continuing to move forward with me on its hood, whimpering. What I later discovered was that I impacted the windshield with enough force to destroy it and was subsequently hurled 20 feet down the road. I remember crashing head first on the asphalt, shattering my bike helmet.

What happened next was nothing short of amazing.

As if guided by an invisible director, people descended on the scene from every bearing. Although conscious, I was — needless to say — confused. I couldn't tell in which direction I was facing, nor from where the voices came, but I could discern individuals coordinating to direct traffic away from me. I heard cell phones click to life from those calling emergency services. Strangers ran to assist me, and one gentleman — an angel as far as I'm concerned — took my head in his hands to hold me still to prevent further injury, his calm reassuring voice a comfort unlike anything I can remember. With my head cradled in his grip, I knew I could "let go." Even though there was no major pain, I was moaning, more out of fear. I wanted to sit up to survey what damage had been done to me but this God-send of a man insisted I be still and he held me firm. He assured me help was coming and he would take care of me until then. The EMTs arrived within seconds, as did the fire department, and police. I felt embarrassed by all the commotion I was causing, and by blocking a major highway, but no one seemed bothered. Everyone was focused on helping me.

Someone asked if I was okay.

I quipped, "You mean aside from the obvious?"

He laughed; I cannot say how much that meant. That was a hint of normalcy and I so needed it. While the EMTs checked me out and loaded me into the ambulance, I couldn't help but crack wise. It might not have been the traditional platform for a comedian but — what can I say — when the entertainment bug bites, you just gotta go with it.

The doctor who discharged me later called me the "Man of Steel." He said, "For a 57-year old guy to take the impact you took and be able to walk out of this hospital on your own power means you're either living right, or someone's looking after you — or both." (He also said the helmet saved my life.)

There has been an amazing outpouring of concern for me since the news got out. Everyone asks how I feel. When I woke up today, I realized I had aches in places where I did not even know I had places so my answer is consistent, "Sore and Grateful." This could have ended with countless other outcomes and with so much more pain and suffering than I am enduring today. As many have pointed out (like I don't know), I could have died. Yet none of those happened; none; just some abrasions, sprains, and contusions.

I am lucky beyond calculation.

As importantly, if it wasn't for the kindness of strangers and the professionalism of the first responders, I'm not sure what would be today. All I know for sure is that I am indeed blessed, and I am reminded yet again that none of us exist in isolation. We come together to help each other and from that action, we become our own better angels. We are benevolent, caring, magnificent beings who — when push comes to shove — will do the good thing.

I don't ever want to go through that again; that probably goes without saying. However in some unlikely manner, the faith it has given me, the hope it has provided me, and the reminder of what really matters has sincerely made yesterday one of the best days in my life. I am grateful to everyone who helped more than I can ever express.

God bless you.

OBSERVATIONS AFTER AN ACCIDENT

This is my 312th column, putting a period on six years. These thoughts I share every week do not have a "mission statement" or goal per se; however, I always aspire to use the privilege of this space (and your time) to inspire, uplift, and to be supportive in whatever way I can. If I am also able to generate a laugh or two in the process, that makes it all the better. However, whatever my topic, I attempt to tie these dispatches into what I consider the "big picture;" that each of us possesses the ability to be who we wish to be. Whether we indeed want to drop a few pounds, improve our relationships, or just smile more often; the solutions lie not in our actions but in our thoughts, those sparkling connections firing day in and day out between our synapses.

Let's take that concept a little deeper, shall we?

Our thoughts — to a large extent — are altered by our feelings. If I am angry or sad, my thoughts will be unlike when I am happy or excited. Upbeat folks are more inclined to venture down new avenues than depressed folks; who will lean toward stagnation; both of these due in large extent to underlying emotions. Therefore, it makes sense — at least to me — that the more I accentuate the positive, the more I engage in new behaviors.

Why don't we do that more often? It's not that difficult really.

Underneath these thoughts and their triggering feelings lie beliefs. By example, if I believe that life is painful, it's much more difficult to modify my emotions to find the positive than if I believe life is glorious. Since we are always looking to validate our beliefs, we find "proof" of them wherever we look. One who believes life stinks will uncover countless examples as evidence. Whereby, one who loves life will find an equal number shoring up her philosophy. In effect, what you seek generates emotional responses, altering your thoughts, leading to different actions, adjusting the outcome of your life. Change your observations; change your life.

What I have personally observed since my bike accident is a tremendous outpouring of love, support, and good wishes from people I do and do not know. Where I live has some drawbacks; I won't deny it. Yet, it is also populated with the most astounding, assorted, diversity of magnificent individuals.

Here's where beliefs come home to roost. I trust that people the planet over — while not identical — are similar. We rise in the morning hoping to do the best we can, striving to take care of family and to contribute to our communities. We attempt (mostly) to treat others with dignity and respect, and hope that they will do the same with us. We are all fighting — or embracing — the "human condition," coming from and returning to the same place. We are alike.

So, if that is correct, and the citizens of *my* community have been so wondrously caring and compassionate, my beliefs profess that the people where you live are parallel, and that applies no matter where you're reading this. Logically then, if the world is bursting with people who, at their center, support and assist each other, then this planet is a better place than I gave it credit for being.

I cannot prove it of course, but I assure you that it's true. (Besides, it cannot hurt to hold true that belief, can it?)

Again, thank you for the concern. I'm getting better every day.